Resuscitating Nursing:

A Tactical Roadmap for Nurses Who Refuse to Be Silenced

Ashley Grogg MSN-RN, BC-FMP

resuscitatingnursing.com

First Edition

ISBN Paperback 978-1-969036-00-2
ISBN Kindle 978-1-969036-02-6

Cover Photo by Melissa Dewitt Photography

Printed in the United States of America.

Disclaimer:

This book is for educational and informational purposes only. It reflects the personal experiences and opinions of the author and is not intended to serve as legal advice. While every effort has been made to ensure accuracy, no guarantee is made that errors or omissions are not present. Always consult a qualified attorney for legal guidance specific to your situation or jurisdiction.

For Permissions contact info@wtajourney.com

Dedication

This book is dedicated to God, with thanksgiving for all the lessons that led me here.

To my loving Husband for his steadfast strength.

To my Children for their patience and grace.

To my Mom for teaching me compassion.

To my Dad for making me tenacious.

To my mentor Dan Thiele.

To my political family: Curt, Mary, John, Angie & Amy.

To Janet Converset, RN, who shaped me as a nurse and tamed my spirit without crushing it.

To Joe O.

To all the nurses before and after me.

To all the patients who have struggled in the system.

Contents

Foreword

This book isn't for the nurse who's just checking boxes and keeping quiet. It's not for the ones towing the line, afraid to make waves.

Resuscitate Nursing is for the nurse who knows deep down they were created for such a time as this.

Ashley Grogg didn't set out to write a book. She set out to answer a calling—one that pulled her into legislative battles, political arenas, and deeply uncomfortable truths. She gave her time, energy, and heart—not for a paycheck, but because she couldn't not do it.

She was called by God. And she obeyed.

Ashley didn't just study policy—she entered the fire. She brings to this work the conviction of someone who's walked through it, the clarity of someone who's done her homework, and the heart of someone who loves this profession enough to fight for it.

This book is a wake-up call for nurses who are ready to rise. It's a voice of encouragement for the ones who just need a little more confidence to step into their courage. Ashley's words speak directly to the remnant—the nurses who see the cracks in the system and know they were born to repair them.

She brings her full, authentic self to these pages—unfiltered, unwavering, and full of grace.

There may not be a lot of you reading this who feel that same fire. But the truth is, it doesn't take a lot to make change. It takes a few nurses with righteous conviction and bold obedience.

If you're holding this book, chances are—you're one of them.

Read it. Let it stir you. Then rise and resuscitate what's been lost.

— Jodi O'Malley, MSN, RN
Founder, Righteous RN and Nurses Out Loud
Federal Whistleblower, Advocate, Educator

Note to the Reader

"Live life when you have it. Life is a splendid gift—
there is nothing small about it."
- Florence Nightingale

Do you remember what it felt like when you became a nurse?

That mix of joy, purpose, and power? For many of us, that's been replaced by exhaustion, despair, and the nagging sense that we're watching the profession—and our patients—slip through the cracks.

This book isn't for the faint of heart.

It's for the nurse who's sick of watching corners get cut, ethics get blurred, and leadership excusing the inexcusable.

It doesn't matter if you work in or out of the hospital.
You don't need a title. You don't need permission.
You *just* need a backbone.
Because making real change in nursing isn't just uncomfortable, it *is* war.

You will be disliked.
You will be dismissed, gaslit, and pressured to "tone it down."
You'll be told to play nice, sit on a committee, or keep the peace, while patients suffer and nurses burn out.

This book is for the nurse who doesn't flinch.
The one who doesn't go looking for a fight, but won't back down when their profession's credibility is crumbling around them.
It's for nurses who are done with performative politics, empty gestures, and slow suicide by compromise.

Nurses at the bedside, in management, or in private practice
Nurses who will not trade moral clarity for popularity or comfort.

Nurses who are willing to be called "difficult" for standing between a patient and harm.

If that's you, keep reading.

Because you're exactly the kind of dangerous this profession needs.

We're not here to make noise.

We're here to Resuscitate Nursing.

1
Nursing Has Changed

"Were there none who were
discontented with what they have,
the world would never reach anything better."
- Florence Nightingale

That title is such a cliche, isn't it? Of course, nursing has changed.

It *SHOULD* change. But we hope that it changes for the better. Changes like improved patient outcomes, decreased risks, and better resources, both human and supplies.

That isn't the reality.

Nursing, largely, has changed for the worse.

Mistakes, overmedication, lack of meaningful patient education, and advocacy that lead to unnecessary procedures, poor staffing, high levels of turnover, increased workplace violence, the loss of nursing autonomy, and nursing ethics.

Have we lost touch with ethics? Are nurses losing their edge? Are they forgetting why they got into the profession in the first place? Are they just there for the paycheck?

No! The answer should be no.

Many nurses have been burned so severely that they have lost the fight for ethics and advocacy. Most choose self-preservation in the face of overwhelming responsibility and abusive relationships with both patients and admin. They feel helpless and even hopeless. They are exhausted and don't know where to begin. We can turn that around. We can restore hope, a sense of agency, healthy boundaries, and even a sense of joy.

Before we go any further, I want to remind you of someone who *never* chose self-preservation when the stakes were high: Florence Nightingale.

Nightingale was not just the "lady with the lamp." She was a revolutionary reformer. She was data-driven, politically savvy, and uncompromising in her pursuit of better care. Her legacy wasn't built on comfort; it was forged in courage, clarity, and conviction. She walked straight into broken systems and demanded they change. **She is proof that one nurse can make a difference, and that difference can have a lasting impact across generations.**

Rather than becoming exasperated and throwing our hands up, we must take this opportunity to follow Florence's lead, light our lamps, and **RESUSCITATE NURSING**.

Feeling numb, drained, or stuck in survival mode isn't brokenness. It is the natural fallout of moral injury, learned helplessness, and a *silent curriculum* that taught you to prioritize others no matter the cost. Nursing culture and the healthcare industry praise those who sacrifice the most, quietly modeling martyrdom as professionalism. Over time, repetitive self-sacrifice trains you to stop asking for help, stop expecting better, and forget that your needs matter.

We are resuscitating nursing, so we must identify and correct the invisible curriculum being taught in our profession. It starts with a quiet rebellion, with you, with simple boundaries, and with saying, "Enough is enough."

The Problem

Addressing the knowledge deficit around advocacy and policy change cannot rely on clinical time alone.

Professional advocacy is not just an "add-on" to bedside care. It is part of the broader responsibility we carry as nurses to protect and promote the health of our profession and our patients. This is a professional commitment beyond the clock, pursued not because it is easy or convenient, but because it is essential.

If nurses remain politically disengaged, our silence becomes complicity in systems that harm both caregivers and patients. This section is about reclaiming that power, not piling on another task, but awakening a deeper purpose.

So, what are the challenges?

1. ***Knowledge Deficit*** related to effective nursing advocacy and policy change, secondary to being overwhelmed, exhausted, and lacking accessible guidance on effective change-making in healthcare.

Goal: Nurses will demonstrate increased knowledge and confidence in advocacy efforts and policy engagement within 3–6 months through structured education and peer support.

Nursing Interventions:

1. **Provide structured education and mentorship** on nursing advocacy, including policy change strategies, grassroots mobilization, and effective communication with decision-makers.

2. **Develop and distribute resources** such as guides, checklists, and case studies on successful nursing advocacy efforts.

3. **Facilitate peer support networks** where nurses can share experiences, challenges, and strategies to increase confidence and reduce feelings of isolation.

4. **Support time management and prioritization** skills to help nurses balance professional duties with advocacy efforts without becoming overwhelmed.

5. **Create professional development opportunities** related to nursing policy and leadership.

2. ***Moral Distress*** related to ethical conflicts in patient care and professional practice secondary to institutional policies, loss of nursing autonomy, and systemic barriers to safe, ethical nursing care.

Goal: Nurses will feel supported and equipped to voice concerns and engage in ethical decision-making processes within their organizations.

Nursing Interventions:

1. **Create a safe space for open discourse** where nurses can discuss ethical concerns without fear of retaliation.

2. **Educate nurses on institutional and legislative processes** to empower them to advocate for changes that support ethical practice and nursing autonomy.

3. **Develop a framework for ethical decision-making** to guide nurses in addressing moral dilemmas in practice.

4. **Encourage the creation and participation in grassroots professional nursing organizations** focusing on advocacy and policy reform.

5. **Promote resilience-building strategies** such as mindfulness, peer support, and professional counseling to mitigate the emotional toll of moral distress.

3. ***Risk of Burnout*** related to sustained engagement in nursing activism and advocacy, secondary to emotional labor, resistance from leadership, and the prolonged effort required to drive systemic change.

Goal: Nurses will implement sustainable strategies for self-care, boundary setting, and peer collaboration within 3–6 months to reduce emotional fatigue and prevent burnout related to advocacy.

Nursing Interventions:

1. **Encourage self-care,** including adequate rest, physical activity, and stress management techniques.

2. **Teach boundary-setting skills** to help nurses balance activism with personal and professional responsibilities.

3. **Promote delegation and teamwork** to distribute advocacy efforts among a larger group and prevent individual overburden.

4. **Provide mental health support and peer debriefing sessions** to address emotional fatigue and sustain motivation.

5. **Celebrate small victories and progress** to maintain morale and reinforce the impact of ongoing advocacy efforts.

"If nurses recognize their power to do good and untether the strings of bureaucracy, there is no stopping us." - Ashley Grogg

If the first care plan sparked a flash of rage, this part is for you.

Let's be clear: this isn't about blaming nurses. It's not about piling on more work during an already impossible shift. It's about resuscitating a piece of our professional responsibility that has been quietly stripped away—or never taught to begin with.

That's why this book exists. Nurses feel helpless. They're taking hit after hit, and nothing's getting better. But it's not because we don't care. It's because nurses aren't being equipped with the tools and feel they must wait for permission to act.

This is the missing piece: understanding how to advocate for change, not just in a hospital room, but in the systems that shape those rooms.

Yes, it's going to take effort outside of work hours. And no, it's not fair. That can be hard to swallow, but it goes beyond our careers. The implications are severe for nurses yet to come and, more importantly, their patients. Those patients may include you or your loved ones.

Sometimes text isn't quite as effective in communicating my humor. I hope you got a chuckle at my corniness- but yeah, I went there. I care-planned our profession, because when systems fail, nurses assess the situation, identify the root causes, and intervene. That's precisely what this is: a care plan, not for a patient, but to resuscitate nursing.

I. AM. NOT. ASHAMED.

While I did it in part for giggles, the process works. Once I started care planning, I couldn't stop.

The stark reality of our situation hit me like a ton of bricks as I worked. The benefit of objectifying the issue is that creating a black-and-white illustration helps frame it for what it truly is. Broken. Even though I was trying to be silly, the care plans I created certainly caught my attention and made me realize how much we need to resuscitate our profession.

The question is, how?

Removing Fear & Knowing What To Do

Knowing where to start and what to do is often a deterrent to making change. Leaving the security of being the expert is terrifying.

This is precisely what I experienced when I went from nursing into political activism. I felt God was thrusting me into an area I knew nothing about. A place where I had to humble myself and acknowledge it would be quite a while before I became proficient, let alone assume the role of expert and mentor I had become accustomed to in nursing.

Being wrong is scary.

The only thing worse than being wrong is abandoning something you love and cherish. I love and cherish my profession, but am disheartened by what it has become.

I will not back down.

I will not go away.

We will resuscitate our profession.

The beautiful thing is, our nursing knowledge and processes give us a tactical advantage when assuming a new and scary role. I have relied heavily on the same skills I used for nursing to help me work effectively in politics. After all, it is just another form of advocacy.

While creating the nursing diagnosis above was more a point of humor, the nursing diagnosis above perfectly illustrates how our nursing skills give us a unique advantage for making change. We do it all the time, just on an individualized level.

Creating nursing diagnoses and implementing interventions will help you along your advocacy journey for our profession. You will read more about this later. For now, I want to focus on teaching you how to utilize your nursing skills to alleviate the fear and confusion associated with making changes.

We must remember how, in this instance, our profession is our patient, and it is our responsibility to make it healthy again. More on this later…

Informed Decision-Making In Advocacy

There are risks associated with every action or inaction we take. We continually conduct micro-risk benefit analyses to inform our next steps. It is a fact of life.

"Should I turn on red?"

"Can I sleep for another five minutes without being late for work?"

"Do I move across the country for my dream job?"

Some of these questions have immediate impacts. Others may not be realized until much later. Regardless, our decisions will impact our future, good or bad. Becoming an advocate for nursing will not be any different.

You will likely be disliked, scorned, and ridiculed, and you may even risk losing your job simply by acting on the brokenness of our profession and restoring moral and ethical behavior. The medical system is complex. There are many players with varying stakes, including those who have a vested interest in the status quo.

These players will be present if you work "inside" or "outside" of the system. It truly doesn't matter. We have to understand the political machine behind the problems.

Hospital systems prioritize both their bottom line and their public image. *You will be on their radar as soon as you become an effective agent of change that impacts them.*

When you are effective, **medical associations** that visualize themselves as advocates for professionals may see you as a threat, and characterize you as overstepping your bounds, or even "ruining" things for others. Some medical associations view advocacy or lobbying as a lucrative aspect of their work. Being effective makes you a threat to their funding, reputation, and stability. Others find great financial benefit in the next training or service offered to mask the symptoms of our broken system. Do not generalize and assume all associations are bad. Use your discernment and critical thinking skills to sort them out.

Other professionals will also notice as you gain traction and make changes. Don't be surprised when they are not appreciative. They may be scared by the threats from hospital systems and medical associations. They might even be told things like, "If (your organization) doesn't stop, then (threat). You must ensure they know what they do is detrimental to (institution/patients/morale)." Other professionals may harbor guilt or shame over wrong actions or methods, and accepting change would validate those feelings. Or worse yet, they might be afraid of having to do the work and, therefore, resist or even sabotage your efforts.

Any of these groups may also solicit the help of others to attempt to dissuade you from continuing your mission. They may include friends, peers, management, members of the public, politicians, lawyers, and more.

Their attempts to thwart your efforts will range from aggressive to hateful and downright vindictive. However, don't be fooled by flattery, promotion, or power. These are tools to neutralize you. Mainly because those promotions and power often come with restrictive strings and control. If you want to keep the power they give you, you will have to play by their rules. We will discuss this in more depth later.

That all sounds a lot like politics, doesn't it?

Politics & Nursing Advocacy?

Politics invades nearly everything because it is "the science or art of governing". Naturally, there is an order; there are leaders and followers. There is always structure, management, and leadership when working for an organization. Due to those factors, we see political motives and actions in nearly every aspect of our work.

Whether we like it or not, the healthcare system is intertwined with politics, not only because of the act of governing, but also due to actual Government and political involvement related to insurance, Medicare, Medicaid, and the legal regulations placed on entities and individuals working in healthcare. Regardless of whether you realize it, simply by being a member of the medical community, you *are* involved in politics, and they impact you, your patients, and your decisions.

Isn't it time we used politics to advance moral and ethical decision-making, in addition to policies?

Motivation

Let's be honest, this problem is BIG.

It is much bigger than you and me.

It is bigger than the organizations we work for.

It is bigger than the corporations that own our organizations.

The odds are NOT in our favor. Powerful forces are arrayed against us. However, we are unstoppable with dedicated nurses around the country taking action and making consistent changes in their hospitals, communities, and states.

You must find your motivation to remain consistent and persevere through the obstacles.

Why are you willing to face insurmountable odds?

The patients? Dedication to your profession? Fear of what the future will hold? To prevent or heal your moral injury?

Why will you persevere despite attacks, slander, threats, and "losing" opportunities for promotion? What will carry you through the hard days? Who are you going to turn to for support?

Once you have found your motivation, the rest is relatively simple.

I am committed to providing you with a clear outline and the necessary tools to achieve success. The next several chapters will walk you through detailed information, but here are the basics.

1. Politics 101, (How politics really works)
2. Identifying the Problem
3. Prioritizing the Best Battle
4. Building Your Team
5. Strategic Communication
6. Mobilization

Don't miss out on the free worksheets over at wtajourney.com/rnbook, better yet, get the full Resuscitating Nursing Workbook & Field Manual on Amazon, if you haven't yet. It has all the worksheets plus so much more. You can also find a network of nurses by joining the private membership community and monthly mentorship where I will support you in developing action plans, take problems head-on, and answer the questions no one else seems to have answers to.

2
Politics 101

*"I attribute my success to this—
I never gave or took any excuse."*
- Florence Nightingale

You didn't become a nurse to play politics, but politics plays a role in every part of your job.

Staffing ratios? That's policy.

Hospital funding? That's policy.

Insurance reimbursements, scope of practice, and patient rights?

All policies...

Politics always drives policies, whether hospital rules, workplace regulations, or national healthcare laws. Every decision that shapes nursing practice comes from a political process.

Laws passed by politicians dictate everything from hospital funding and staffing ratios to licensing requirements and patient care standards. But it's not just lawmakers pulling the strings. Big players, including pharmaceutical companies, insurance providers, hospital associations, and other special interest groups, pour millions into lobbying to shape policies that serve their interests, often at the expense of medical professionals and the patients they serve.

> ***Pro Tip:*** Lobbying is the act of persuading a politician or government official to take a specific action. Special interest groups often hire professionals to deliver targeted messaging, and sometimes propaganda, to influence policies or regulations that benefit their industry.

These same groups are in play within hospitals, too. Policies aren't just about what's best for care; government regulations, legal risks, and financial incentives heavily influence them. Patient care may not even be the highest priority on the list, even in so-called non-profit entities.

The bottom line here is that *NO ONE IS EXEMPT FROM POLITICAL INTERFERENCE.*

We have all watched how this has happened in the hospital system. There is a stark contrast between what healthcare was ten to twenty years ago and what it is now.

The industry mindset has not only taken root but has also completely changed the way healthcare is delivered. Cookie-cutter medicine is employed with a focus on automated protocols, a dependency on disconnected specialization silos, the idolization of computerized documentation in the name of portability, and an increasing financial force being used to ensure diagnoses are "treated the same," even when it isn't best for the patient.

We are up against the big dogs. Right now, it feels futile.

I can relate.

When I was working in the hospital, I tried to fight.

My manager tried to fight.

Sadly, I watched as the system consumed her. She is still in various positions, and she is trying to fight the good fight the best way she knows how. God bless her.

I worked my way up the "ladder" into a quasi-management position as a "data coordinator," developing the heart failure program along with some fantastic and compassionate people, including the manager who would go to bat for us.

Our efforts were in vain due to stonewalling by unphased hospital leadership, much higher than her.

Our hospital was chronically short-staffed, went on hiring freezes, and experienced a high turnover rate.

I advocated, joined all the committees, and tried to play the game.

It wasn't enough.

A Missed Opportunity

At one point, our hospital got a new CEO. Young, energetic, and full of hope. He walked into the lion's den full of nurses who had been used and abused. They were angry and short-tempered.

Needless to say, as he made promises about staffing and other issues, he was brutally called out and lambasted by the nurses he promised to help.

At that moment, I stood up. I asked my peers to give the man an opportunity since he was just arriving. I also warned that I would not defend him again if he failed to keep his promises.

A year or more passed, and staffing was worse than ever before. From the stage of the hospital auditorium, he had the audacity to point out the shortcomings of nursing while completely ignoring the glaring issues related to critical staffing shortages, failure to hire, and abysmally low retention rates.

I stood up and reminded him of when he first came to the hospital. I reminded him of how I had defended him after he had made promises about improving staffing, and how it was the root of every issue he dared criticize nursing about.

With bold confidence, as he perched on a stool, one leg tucked onto the rugs and the other outstretched, he looked at me and suggested, "Well, I think maybe you should join a committee."

Before he finished the word "committee," the director of cardiac services, my boss's boss, sitting behind him, had placed her hand on his shoulder. In an embarrassed and hushed voice still audible to the crowd, she stated, "She is on every committee." The CEO's body stiffened, shifting from his comfortable position to the edge of his chair with both feet planted on the floor as his face turned bright red. He moved to a different question quickly.

I missed an opportunity that day.

I was confrontational, and I was brave. I asserted facts and called on him to act on his promises.

That's accountability, right?!?

It wasn't enough.

NOTHING CHANGED, except he made every effort to divert to a different route if he saw me coming.

I clearly made an impact, but nothing changed.

Why didn't he listen to my facts?

Why didn't he live up to his promises?

Why couldn't they understand something so simple?

Morally, how could he be so nasty to the people who were busting their backs for him?

Now, I know it was political pressure. He was facing extreme political pressure from corporate officers who held his reputation and job in their hands. Looking back, I wish I had known then what I know now.

Everything went on, business as usual. Staffing continued to be abysmally low while management piled more tasks onto the backs of nurses. I felt like I was failing my patients and fellow nurses. There was no way to "fix it". I had continuously made my observations known and did my best to be a "part of the solution," but it wasn't good enough.

The most painful part was knowing that the patients were still paying the price for all of it. They were missing baths, call lights went off for what felt like forever, and I knew significant errors were happening. I know of at least two, if not three, preventable deaths that had been swept under the rug.

When we did have staff, they would be "floated" out to other departments with critical staffing needs. As the charge nurse, I struggled to keep our nurses on the unit because we had "tripled" ICUs with no charge nurse. This was LONG before COVID.

Being in that environment was sucking the soul from my body. I knew we weren't providing the care our patients deserved. As a "coordinator," I knew I was creating policies that staff couldn't reasonably carry out due to patient ratios. Just by doing my job, I was failing the nurses as much as I was the patients. I was contributing to their struggle.

Can you relate?

Have you been in a similar situation?

What would you have done differently?

A Different Way

I commanded a presence, called out the CEO, and had the knowledge and the experience. I was even "on every committee" – none of it was enough, and none of it mattered.

If I knew then what I know now, I would have CONTINUED to apply pressure to that CEO. I would have leveraged the largest number of employees in the hospital, the nurses.

It wasn't that I wasn't willing. It was that I didn't know there was a different way. I don't want that to happen to you. I am going to teach you what I have learned since.

Years later, after leaving that hospital and experiencing more of the same while working as a nurse in the insurance industry, I left Western medicine with a broken heart, as I watched the moral backbone of my profession disintegrate under the industrial mindset.

I began working in advocacy and knew politics was going to be the way I could make change. My personal experience had been limited to education. Education alone isn't enough to make a change.

There was only one problem.

I was "politically apathetic."

Some of my apathy was related to the fact that I didn't know how the government worked. My parents never spoke about politics. If I am being candid, I slept through government and economics in high school. So aside from what I could remember from School House Rock's "I'm Just a Bill," I didn't understand how the government worked at all.

This was incredibly humbling for me. I was always someone who knew "all the things" and was often a point of reference for others.

My own attitude was the most significant barrier to progress. I hated politics. I am a no-nonsense farm kid. I grew up expecting that you did the right thing, did it well, and ALWAYS finished the job.

I am not good at kissing backside, playing games, or beating around the bush. If I don't say it, you can and will read exactly what I am thinking all over my face.

Politics was precisely the opposite. Or so I thought.

An acquaintance suggested that I attend an all-day political seminar, and I thought she was NUTS. I literally laughed out loud.

"Could you imagine me in a room with a bunch of suits? That won't end well."

I signed up for the class, paid 40ish bucks, and prepared to be disappointed.

The class was scheduled for February 1st. My expectations were LOW.

They were so low that I said yes when my friend asked if I would help her clean her Grandpa's barn. I told her about the class and that I would be leaving early. I suggested we meet in town for an early lunch, and then we would get to work.

For a frame of reference, Grandpa's barn is a steel building without heat or insulation. *It doesn't have heat*, and we live in northern Indiana, where the average temperatures in January and February are in the 20s and 30s.

I'm not sure if I need to repeat it, but my expectations for this political seminar were LOW. I planned on leaving the class at the ten am break so we could still have plenty of time to clean the barn that day, in the frigid cold.

The morning of the class, I was kicking myself. Why was I driving an hour away early on a bitterly cold Saturday morning?

I arrived at the address listed. It was an old stone church in the middle of nowhere, and the gravel crunched under my tires as I pulled in. I thought, "This is a sketch," as I grabbed my notebook and headed in.

I met two other women I had previously known, but only through the internet. We joked about the insanity we were embarking on and settled into our seats. I never imagined what would unfold that day.

The class wasn't quite what I expected. A tall, lumberjack-looking man with red hair and a fiery personality to match led the class. His wife sat calmly near him, knitting as he lectured like a general leading his men into battle.

It was iconic and so perfect.

During that first segment of the class, I learned that being successful in politics isn't about being politically correct, playing the name game, or even being the richest in the room.

I learned I could be honest and hold people accountable for their broken promises, and NONE of it involved the things I thought politics entailed.

You have to know the game, but don't have to play it. AND you can be brutally honest the entire time. Well, almost the whole time.

This method of politics doesn't just allow "bullying the bully". It prioritizes it.

They taught me that I could be myself, hold my personal standards, unapologetically set those exact expectations for others, and make a difference.

They also taught me politics is simply a numbers game, and that number is FAR less than I would have ever imagined.

I'm going to say that again- POLITICS IS A NUMBERS GAME. But more on this later.

I was hooked. I was in. I was on the edge of my seat, taking more notes than the teacher's pet, until suddenly, the instructor informed us that we were running behind but would be taking a short break since it was after ten.

I was shaken. How had the time gone so quickly?

There was no way I was going to leave. Without cell service in the church's basement, I ran outside and called my friend from the cold.

She laughed as I apologized and explained that I was going to stay in the class. I repeated myself a couple of times, letting her know I wouldn't be joining her. She didn't believe me.

First of all, it was uncharacteristic for me to cancel, but even more unbelievable that I would cancel to STAY with political junkies at a seminar. She followed up around lunch, thinking I was kidding, but I wasn't.

So, what did I learn that took me from politically apathetic to on fire and ready to make a difference?

Tactics

What I learned that day was life-changing for sure. Within a week of that class, I was sitting in an attorney's office completing paperwork for a non-profit social welfare advocacy group.

Since then, I have successfully applied those basics and expanded my knowledge through education and, most of all, experience. Five years later, a few strangers I met in that class still stand beside me, acting as mentors and some of the best friends I could ask for.

To summarize what I learned-

Regardless of whether they are elected by the citizens or hired by corporations to run a hospital, politicians will all buckle when you find the right buttons.

The best part is, these tactics are effective anywhere you use them.

Politicians and "C-Suite" types (think CEOs, CFOs, etc.) are the same. The pressure points might differ slightly, but they will generally respond similarly.

From this point on, I will refer to elected officials and "C-Suite" types as politicians. If I intend to differentiate, I will make a specific delineation. Sometimes, the way you approach people and your process of informed decision-making will differ depending on the distinction. So, note that when I use something more specific than "politician," I speak about those particular groups.

To create meaningful change, you cannot rely on simply educating politicians.

Politicians are not motivated by facts, reason, or heartfelt pleas for better patient care.

They respond to political pressure.

They respond to political pain.

They respond to the real threat of losing their positions.

Their position is their power, and they have a singular goal- STAY IN POWER. All of the decisions they make revolve around their political survival. Legislators and elected officials balance between the lobbyists and their constituents; if they believe the constituents to be more forgiving, they will 100% go with the lobbyist every time.

Administrators walk the line between what the corporate office and shareholders are saying and how antsy the staff is. If they believe the staff will continue to take the brunt of the abuse and get the job done, they will use and abuse them to execute the wishes of the corporate office.

Who do you think my CEO was more afraid of, the singular nurse who once defended him, or the corporate office that is threatening him with his job and reputation?

If you guess the corporate office, you would be right.

To shift that power dynamic, I would have needed NUMBERS.

I would have needed an army. But more on this later.

There Is More Than One Way to Have Political Influence

There is the direct path, which is becoming an elected official or administrator. There is also an indirect path, sometimes referred to as an "informal leader."

In the farm world, we call informal leaders the "boss cow."

When she bellows- all the other cows respond. It's a real thing, I promise...

We have all seen these in our units. It is the nurse who doesn't hold any formal leadership position. But when things get shaken up or a new policy or therapy is introduced, everyone, including leadership, is watching to see how the "boss cow" will respond.

This can create a problematic situation. Sometimes, leadership will try to persuade the "boss cow" into early adoption because they know that if they have the "boss cow," most of the unit will follow along without much ruckus.

Later, we will discuss "having a seat at the table" and how offers, promotions, decision-making capabilities, and special committees can serve as a means of co-opting or limiting the power of the informal leader. Politicians use this tactic because being granted "special access" can be revoked and viewed as a punishment for not following along with the change. Leadership knows if the "boss cow" isn't having it- EVERYONE will have doubts, regardless of how good the change is.

This informal leadership creates an interesting dynamic because, unless co-opted, the "boss cow" is only accountable to their own morals and those who choose to follow them, unlike the direct path, which is responsible to multiple groups. For example, the CEO is accountable to his direct management, the shareholders, the management below him, and the individuals within the company.

Taking the indirect path for an employee may be risky to your employment. We will discuss ways to safeguard your employment, but honestly, there are no guarantees. You must decide how far you will push and at what point it is better to move on from an organization. Entry-level or "low-level" employees are at less risk than someone in a supervisory capacity.

A final cautionary note- as nurses, we must never forget that our duty is to keep the patient safe. Ethically, we are bound to advocate for them and ensure they have the best possible outcomes. In your advocacy, do not become so hasty that you use a patient as a means to an end or jeopardize their safety in any way.

Pushing Political Pain Points to Elicit Change

Politicians of all kinds react strongly when you push the right buttons. These fall into a few key categories. I will list them below for a quick review, and then we will dive into each area individually.

1. **Public Embarrassment**
2. **Mobilization of Voters/Employees (Nurses & Allies)**
3. **Financial Disruption**
4. **Forced Transparency & Accountability**
5. **Threaten Their Job Security**
6. **Legal, Board, or Accreditation Investigations**

How Nurse Advocates Can Create Public Embarrassment

Public embarrassment is one of the most effective ways to push hospital administration into action. Administrators rely on maintaining a polished reputation.

Just remember, this isn't about their personal reputation. It is their professional reputation. Be sure that the information you are using is factual. You always want to "bring the receipts" so that you do not face legal concerns. When the reputation is threatened, they often move quickly to protect it. Here's how nurse advocates can apply this tactic:

- **Leverage Patient and Family Testimonies:**
  Educate patients or their families about self-advocacy, including sharing their experiences in public forums, hospital reviews, or news reports.

Rationale: Nothing damages a hospital's reputation faster than real patient horror stories.

- **Blast Them in the Media:**
Write op-eds, letters to the editor, or coordinate press coverage on patient safety issues, staffing ratios, or administrative negligence, including photos, copies, or other evidence. Evaluate the risk and determine if anonymous reports are best. Social media outcry may also be effective.
Rationale: If bad press starts circulating, the administration will scramble to save face.

- **Call Them Out in Public Meetings:**
Attend board meetings, town halls, or public hospital events and ask direct, pointed questions about unsafe conditions.
Rationale: Put them on the spot where they can't dodge accountability.

- **Rally Community Support:**
Mobilize local organizations or patient advocacy groups to protest hospital policies or demand administrative change
Rationale: Public pressure makes it clear that inaction is not an option.

- **Expose Conflicts of Interest or Mismanagement:**
Research and publish information on how hospital executives prioritize profits over patient care, such as executive bonuses amid staffing shortages.
Rationale: Nothing makes an administrator panic faster than being exposed for hypocrisy.

How Nurse Advocates Can Mobilize Employees & Allies

Numbers matter. As I sat in that political seminar, this fact caught my attention. I knew numbers mattered. However, I didn't realize that the "number needed to treat" was much smaller than I had ever imagined.

The seminar laid it out beautifully, explaining that elections aren't won by 50% plus one. They then revealed that the number of votes truly in play in most situations slowly diminishes to a whopping 3% plus one.

The lecture explained that not everyone can vote, which cuts down the population you need to reach. Some players always vote a certain way. In politics, it is people who will always vote red or blue. These people are NOT who you want to talk to or focus the majority of your energy on.

Think about those people in your facility. There are always people who will remain apathetic, who won't take a stand regardless of the circumstances. They might be travelers, PRN, or other positions with little to no "buy-in". Some are ready to retire, losing the will or interest to create change, and others are just paycheck collectors. For our purpose, none of them has a vote…

The next group that can be eliminated from your mobilization efforts is those who will always side with leadership and management. This group will "vote" the way they always do. DO NOT WASTE YOUR TIME ARGUING WITH THOSE WHO WILL NEVER AGREE WITH YOU.

Don't ignore those who will always rebel against the system, but you shouldn't waste your time convincing those who already agree with you anyway. Let them know what you are doing, invite them to join your efforts, and provide them with *actionable* items. They will be easy conversions; let them help you educate and mobilize others.

In politics, what ends up being left "in play" is about 6% of the population; so to win, candidates or advocacy groups only need to win 3% plus 1. I don't think this has been studied in healthcare; however, these tactics have been employed in various political bodies, ranging from nursing homes and HOAs to state and federal politics. Why would hospitals be any different?

If the theory holds, that means you only need to find your 3% plus 1.

Can you find 3 out of every 100 nurses to lock arms with you? Look around the hospital at the number of nurses- this will help you figure out your total and 3%. Your focus will be on gathering a small team, then identifying those "wild cards" who haven't committed to a side or chosen to give up their votes.

When hospital administrators see nurses, staff, and allies uniting, they are forced to listen. The numbers game is one of the most important parts of advocacy and political activism.

If I were to reflect on how I could have handled the situation at my old hospital, I know I could have quickly mobilized the nurses who witnessed what I said that day.

I should have waited outside those doors and started asking people if they wanted to make a change. I should have started gathering those who agreed with me and been able to channel their frustration into meaningful actions.

Here's how to mobilize effectively:

- **Organize Staff Petitions:**
  Circulate petitions demanding changes, collecting signatures from nurses, staff, and allies to show broad support.
  Rationale: *A united workforce is harder to ignore. PLUS, this helps you identify your 3% and communicate with them in the future. So, be sure to collect contact info.*

- **Encourage Staff to Speak Out:**
  Train staff on how to voice concerns publicly, whether in news stories, at board meetings, or otherwise.
  Rationale: *More voices = more pressure. The SBAR format works beautifully.*

- **Leverage Patients & Families:**
  Encourage community members to join the cause, emphasizing how administrative failures impact care.
  Rationale: *Public outcry = fast-track to change.*

- **Use Social Media to Organize & Inform:**
  Create private nurse advocacy groups to coordinate strategies, updates, and actions.
  Rationale: *Keep everyone informed and engaged. These groups are never private, so ensure everyone maintains professionalism.*

How Nurse Advocates Can Use Financial Disruption

Hospitals care about one thing above all: their bottom line. Stakeholders get angry if the finances are failing. Corporate officers will quickly take notice if they suspect even a hint of financial loss. If patient safety concerns threaten revenue, administrators act fast. Here's how to leverage financial disruption:

- **Expose the Cost of Turnover:**
  Highlight the financial loss from high nurse turnover due to poor working conditions. These costs may include man-hours, benefits, extra costs associated with travelers, and much more.
  Rationale: When the administration sees the cost of losing skilled nurses, they'll be more inclined to address concerns.

- **Publicize Lawsuits & Payouts:**
  Draw attention to malpractice suits and settlements resulting from administrative failures.
  Rationale: Show how poor policies are costing them big money.

- **Target Donors & Sponsors:**
  Inform hospital donors about unsafe conditions and encourage them to demand accountability.
  Rationale: Money talks; if donors pull funding, changes happen.

Some of these areas may be more difficult if you do not have access to sensitive information. If you do, this could be a more precarious endeavor for you. It might be better to develop relationships where one person can provide the details and another can expose it without revealing the source.

How Nurse Advocates Can Use Forced Transparency & Accountability

Administrators thrive in secrecy and plausible deniability. Forcing them into the light makes evasion impossible. This is an area where I have recognized my own shortcomings. I know I don't continue to force transparency and accountability like I should. It is easy to mention something once and then drop it. When we are talking about ensuring accountability, this is an ONGOING process.

I am sure that other nurses also fall into that same trap. It isn't because we don't want accountability, but because we expect others to have the same autonomous drive to correct course and fix a problem once it is identified.

I hate to break it to you… That is NOT how most of the world works. As you work towards transparency and accountability, you must remember to be persistent and keep hammering home the same points until you achieve the desired change. Then, once change happens, you must keep pressing on the issue to ensure the change isn't temporary.

Often, when I speak about politicians, I use analogies related to correcting children's behavior. You must be persistent, make frequent reminders, and stay the course because as soon as you look the other way, they will be right back to their same old antics.

Here's how to demand transparency and accountability:

- **Demand Public Data on Staffing & Patient Outcomes:** Request records on staffing ratios, patient wait times, and incident reports through official channels or public records requests (if applicable).
  Rationale: If they refuse, they have something to hide; turn up the pressure and expose the refusal.

- **Call for Independent Audits:**
  Push for third-party evaluations of patient safety metrics, financial allocations, or HR practices.
  Rationale: External scrutiny eliminates their ability to manipulate internal reports.

- **Expose Contradictions & Broken Promises:**
  Keep a documented timeline of what was promised versus what has been done and publish discrepancies.
  Rationale: Showing a pattern of deception will mobilize your group and increase pressure, forcing accountability.

- **Require Town Halls or Open Meetings:**
  Insist that leadership hold open forums with staff and patients, where they must answer direct questions.
  Rationale: Making them face the people they are failing increases pressure to act.

- **Publish Internal Policies That Harm Care:**
  Bring to light outdated or unethical policies prioritizing hospital profits over patient safety. Have the solution, or a start to the solution, with evidence-based practices to back them up.
  Rationale: Publicizing these forces immediate reform or damages their credibility.

- **Shine Light on Public Documents:**
  Expose hard truths within publicly available reports or data that rarely receive attention.
  Rationale: This information is readily available and "low hanging fruit." Because it is already public there is little additional risk.

How Nurse Advocates Can Threaten Job Security

Just like politicians, administrators fear losing their positions. Make them feel the heat by creating the perception that their leadership is untenable. The thing about politicians is they talk, they gossip, and they are kind of a "Mean Girls" clique. If an administrator loses control of their facility and subsequently loses their job, they will likely face difficulty finding a replacement position.

Here's how to threaten job security:

- **Expose Scandals or Poor Performance:**
  Research administrators, track records, and bring attention to failures under their leadership, high turnover, lawsuits, complaints, etc., and make them public.
  <u>Rationale:</u> *If they become a liability, the board will replace them.*
- **Mobilize a Vote of No Confidence:**
  Rally nurses and staff to sign a formal declaration of no confidence in hospital leadership.
  <u>Rationale:</u> *A workforce publicly rejecting them weakens their standing with the board and investors.*
- **Apply Pressure to the Hospital Board:**
  Communicate directly with board members and major donors about administrative failures.
  <u>Rationale:</u> *If they believe their investments or reputations are at risk, they will demand leadership changes.*
- **Highlight Financial Mismanagement:**
  Investigate bonuses, executive compensation, and wasteful spending, then expose discrepancies.
  <u>Rationale:</u> *If they are profiting while the hospital struggles, they become expendable.*
- **Encourage Community Leaders to Speak Out:**
  Bring city officials, patient advocacy groups, or religious leaders into the conversation.
  <u>Rationale:</u> *External voices calling for leadership change make it harder for the board to ignore.*

Solid Ground. I am going to risk sounding contradictory here, but there is nuance to all of these tactics, and this, I feel, is especially worth pointing out. There are rare occasions when politicians, administrators, and even CEOs can be allies.

I was talking with a former co-worker about the situation with the CEO in the story above, and I think it is important to share with you what she said, "I stood up for him too, and I think he did try to fulfill [his promises]. But, micromanaging from out-of-state corporate offices caused delays in hiring."

She continued, "I think your interaction about joining a committee was one of many that humbled him. I think he had a lot to learn. I was still on third shift at that time, and he was frequently there late. One night, he came up and looked over the schedule with me, both of us frustrated with the lack of staff. He asked me why we only had five new nurses starting when he had given authorization to hire 12. I told him we simply didn't have enough experienced nurses left to train anymore than that."

Looking back on the past, I still believe that he and my manager were genuinely trying to help. It was difficult to determine what was real and what wasn't in the moment. There were many times when I was frustrated with both of them and saw them as adversaries, yet at other times, I had such deep compassion for them both. (*cont...*)

I can't help but wonder how I could have used a tactic I like to call "solid ground" to collaborate with them. This is an advanced tactic and one with an incredible amount of nuance. There is no script, protocol, or even flowchart I can give. It is a delicate balance of holding them accountable while simultaneously supporting them and elevating their message to those ABOVE them.

If there is one thing that must be clear about providing solid ground, it is that you are not giving them undue credit. You are not making excuses for them. You are not becoming their political mouthpiece to the people.

It gives them a step up, so they can look their supervisor square in the eye. It is being a battering ram at the door of the corporate office. It is allowing them to say, "Look at what I am up against. These nurses are vast in number, well informed, and organized." In effect, they become your political mouthpiece.

I have effectively used this tactic in politics, and I will say, finding an ally like this is difficult, and it is even more challenging to forge a trusting relationship. It's kind of like love; don't go looking for it, it will find you when you least expect it. Use this with caution and slowly build layers of trust.

I also highly recommend discussing this with your mentor to decrease the chance of being taken advantage of. These kinds of allies may wax and wane, drifting in and out of favor. Be sure not to overpromise. Your messaging will also need to be deliberate. That is a lesson for another day, but a quick tip: Focus on the individual's actions and how the *act* of doing was brave, rather than deeming the individual brave. Nuance is important.

How Nurse Advocates Can Use Legal, Board, or Accreditation Investigations

Legal and regulatory scrutiny is one of the fastest ways to force an administration's hand. One of the first steps you need to take is familiarizing yourself with the Nursing Code of Ethics.

In 2025, the American Nurses Association released an updated version of the Code of Ethics for Nurses. I was blown away when I learned how they emphasized the need for nurses to stand in the face of these problems.

The principles in the Nursing Code of Ethics will guide your practice and serve as both a guidepost for general practices and a protective measure for your license. Use them to advocate for your profession and your patients.

Next, familiarize yourself with your nurse practice act and determine to whom you are responsible for reporting concerns. When I was working in the hospital, we made multiple complaints to the Joint Commission on Accreditation. This third party is just another political player and has no real accountability to patients or staff.

In Indiana, nurses are responsible for reporting unsafe practices to the attorney general's office, which handles the licensing of nurses and other medical professionals, as well as to the hospitals or care facilities themselves.

> ***Pro Tip:*** Locate your nurse practice act through the National Council of State Boards of Nursing's website. www.ncsbn.org/npa

If the hospital is known for a specific program, probation, or the loss of an accreditation may be another means of accountability from an outside authority. However, it should not replace that of the appropriate legal authorities.

Here's how to apply this pressure effectively:

- **File Complaints with Accrediting Bodies:**
  Submit detailed reports to organizations or state health departments on hospital violations.
  <u>Rationale:</u> Loss of accreditation is a financial and reputational nightmare for hospitals.

- **Pursue OSHA & Workplace Safety Investigations:**
  Report unsafe working conditions to OSHA or state labor agencies.
  <u>Rationale:</u> Regulatory fines and oversight will force them to act.

- **Encourage Legal Action for Negligence:**
  Educate affected patients on legal resources to explore malpractice or negligence claims.
  *Rationale: The threat of lawsuits forces risk management teams to demand change. *Note, be careful not to place blame or fault; simply and objectively provide education on resources.*

- **Expose Medicare & Medicaid Compliance Violations:**
  Document and report violations of patient care standards that could jeopardize federal funding.
  Rationale: Losing government reimbursements would be catastrophic for hospital finances.

- **Work with Whistleblower Protection Organizations:**
  If administrators retaliate, collaborate with legal groups specializing in whistleblower protections.
  Rationale: Retaliation lawsuits can turn the tables on corrupt leadership.

Knowing When you Pushed the Right Button

Politicians are all very predictable. They have a set group of reactions they will fall back on. Here's how you can gauge the effectiveness of your tactics and mobilization. Politicians:

1. **Ignore You.**
2. **Pretend to Listen.**
3. **Tell you you are Unreasonable.**
4. **Gaslight You.**
5. **Whine.**
6. **Threaten You or Have Others Threaten You.**
7. **Offer a Seat at the Table.**
8. **Take Action Only When Forced.**

We can't let these go without a little more explanation…

At first, the politician or administrator will likely pretend to **ignore you**. In reality, they are paying attention to your efforts. However, they may play it cool at first. Why?

The reason they may pretend to ignore you at first is, in this age of smartphones and social media, most people sadly have the attention span of a gnat.

Add constant understaffed shifts to this mix and plenty of nurses are not going to last very long at their fledgling political efforts. So the administrator is determining whether or not you have the persistence to stay at this pressure campaign for more than a day or two.

If you are **truly being ignored**, you are doing it wrong. You must complete an evaluation and look at each aspect of your plan. Are you targeting the right group? Are you demanding something specific? Are you mobilizing well? How can you take this up a notch? We will discuss these points as we progress through the various steps. Ultimately, if they are ignoring you, you are not a threat.

Once you start making headway, the administration will likely begin by **pretending to listen.** They will listen when you seek them out, they will smile, nod, offer alternatives, and placate you by saying "they are looking into it." Examples might include:

- **The Bureaucratic Stall:**
  "We understand staffing concerns are a priority, and we're forming a task force to explore potential improvements. We'd love your input on this long-term strategy."
  Translation: We'll drag this out with endless meetings until you give up.

- **The "Be Patient" Excuse:**
  "Change takes time, and we are committed to working through these complex issues. Let's plan to reconvene in six months to evaluate progress."
  Translation: We hope you'll get tired of waiting and drop the issue.

- **The Soft Threat:**
  "We want to ensure all perspectives are heard, and a confrontational approach can sometimes slow progress. Let's work together constructively."
  <u>Translation:</u> If you keep pushing, we'll label you as 'difficult' and make your job harder.

Your job is to go in with a specific plan and implement measurable change.

YOU WILL FAIL THIS STEP IF YOU DON'T HAVE AN ACTIONABLE PLAN FOR YOUR MISSION.

If you have a SMART Plan [see Chapter Three], articulate it clearly, demand accountability, and mobilize your army, the administration will escalate to number three on the list to slow you down FAST. The tactic will be to make you feel as if **you are being unreasonable.**

Look out for the following tactics:

- **The Guilt Trip:**
  "We all want the same thing: great patient care. But your approach is making things harder for everyone."
  <u>Translation:</u> Stop pushing so hard, you're making me uncomfortable.

- **The "Mature" Approach:**
  "We need to be professional about this. The best way to make change is through respectful dialogue, not confrontation."
  <u>Translation:</u> If you keep pressing, I'll call you unprofessional.

- **The "We're Making Progress" Line:**
  "We've already made great strides in improving things. We don't want to jeopardize that progress by being too aggressive."
  <u>Translation:</u> Accept tiny changes so I don't have to do more.

- **The "Don't Burn Bridges" Warning:**
  "You don't want to be seen as combative. That could impact your ability to work with leadership in the future."
  <u>Translation:</u> If you keep pushing, I might retaliate.

- **The "We're All in This Together" Plea:**
  "This isn't us vs. them. We need to work as a team to find solutions."
  Translation: *Stop applying pressure, let me stay in control.*

Just a reminder, your mission was never about being liked. It wasn't about getting promoted. It is about doing what is morally right and just for patients and nurses. Your mission is to resuscitate nursing.

If these are your motives, you are not being unreasonable. Your approach must always point back to the facts. This tactic will eliminate their excuses. Using phrases pointing back to why the change is necessary will further frustrate them, and you will likely face one or more of the following tactics.

You may encounter **gaslighting** in the midst of those meetings or when they are trying to get you to sound reasonable. It is a powerful tool used to manipulate and discredit those pushing for change. Administrators may try to make nurse advocates question their own experiences, memories, or judgments.

Here's what that might sound like:

- **The "You're Overreacting" Dismissal:**
  "I think you're taking this too personally. It's not as bad as you're making it seem."
  Translation: *Your concerns are valid, but I need you to doubt yourself so I don't have to address them.*

- **The "That Never Happened" Denial:**
  "We never said that. You must have misunderstood."
  Translation: *We will pretend that reality didn't happen to make you look unreasonable.*

- **The "You're the Only One" Isolation Tactic:**
  "No one else seems to have a problem with this. Maybe you're just looking for issues."
  Translation: *We want you to feel alone so you stop pushing back.*

- **The "You're Not Qualified" Undermining:**
  "You're not in administration, you don't see the full picture."
  <u>Translation:</u> *Your frontline experience doesn't count because it threatens our authority.*

- **The "You Should Be Grateful" Deflection:**
  "You should appreciate what we've already done instead of focusing on what we haven't."
  <u>Translation:</u> *Accept the bare minimum and stop demanding real change.*

Again, if you survive the gaslighting and manipulation and continue pushing for your SMART plan, you will continue to receive different responses from the administration. Their intent will be to get you to go away.

There have been times when I have had multiple of these tactics used against me at once. It is not uncommon for administration to make **excuses and whine** about how difficult you are making things for them or the hospital.

- **The "We Don't Have the Budget" Excuse:**
  "We'd love to do this, but we just don't have the funds right now."
  <u>Translation:</u> *We have money for executive bonuses and PR campaigns, but not for what actually matters.*

- **The "This Isn't a Priority Right Now" Brush-Off:**
  "There are bigger issues we need to focus on first."
  <u>Translation:</u> *We're never going to prioritize this unless you force us to.*

- **The "Change is Hard" Complaint:**
  "This would disrupt too many workflows."
  <u>Translation:</u> *We prefer the broken system because it's easier for us.*

- **The "Shareholder Pressure" Excuse:**
  "We understand your concerns, but implementing this could create challenges with our board and corporate stakeholders."
  <u>Translation:</u> *If shareholders and executives don't like it, patient care and staff wellbeing will always come second.*

You can guarantee that when you are over the target and moving in towards success, you are likely to face **threats**. Administrators are likely to resort to desperate tactics when backed into a corner. Threats may come directly from the administration or through others following orders from the administration.

- **The Career Threat:**
  "You're putting your job at risk by pushing this so hard."
  Translation: Back down, or we'll find a reason to fire you.

- **The Reputation Smear:**
  "People are starting to question your professionalism and motives."
  Translation: We're spreading rumors to isolate and discredit you.

- **The Licensing Threat:**
  "It seems as though you have lost your focus at work. You are preoccupied with this mission. We'd hate to see you jeopardize your license over this."
  Translation: We're implying regulatory trouble if you keep pushing.

- **The Legal Threat:**
  "Some of what you're saying could be considered defamation."
  Translation: We're dangling the possibility of legal action to scare you into silence.

- **The Social Pressure Play:**
  "Other nurses are uncomfortable with your approach."
  Translation: We're using peer pressure to isolate you and break your resolve.

- **The HR Weaponization:**
  "We've had some concerns about your conduct brought to our attention. We would like you to meet with the HR team."
  Translation: We're manufacturing HR complaints to put you on probation or worse.

- **The Passive-Aggressive Scheduling Move:**
  "Due to recent department needs, we've had to adjust your shift schedule."
  Translation: We're making your work life miserable to make you quit.

They may give you **a seat at the table** as a last-ditch effort. Sometimes this is an invitation to a roundtable, a committee meeting, or some other means of placating you to delay further action or even neutralize you completely. You will likely be met with praise and appreciation for advocating for your cause. You may receive sympathetic statements and encouragement such as:

- **The "Empowerment" Trap:**
  "You seem engaged in these issues. Have you considered taking on a leadership role to help improve communication between staff and administration?"
  Translation: If we can co-opt you into the system, you'll be less likely to challenge it.
- **The False Collaboration Approach:**
  "We truly appreciate your passion for patient care, and we'd love to hear more of your concerns in a structured setting. How about joining our advisory committee to help shape solutions together?"
  Translation: We want to keep you busy in a dead-end committee where your influence is diluted.

The most important thing for you to understand about this approach is that as soon as you take your seat at the table, they have control over you.

If they gave you the seat, they can take it away just as fast. You will either be unwilling to give up your bargaining power or will end up so frustrated when they remove you that you slink away with embarrassment from defeat. This often also includes the loss of credibility and respect from your team if you ask them to compromise or back down while bargaining.

Finally, if you stand firm and push the right political buttons, they may begrudgingly give you what you are demanding. Even at this point, you are still not guaranteed victory.

However, you don't often reach this point without first having to trudge through several of the tactics we have discussed. Bottom line: to even have a chance at victory, you must learn how to press these tactics.

Here's the kicker: when enough public pressure builds, politicians and administrators scramble to change course. That means nurses have power if they're willing to use it.

Politics is shaping your profession, whether you engage or not. So the question is: will you sit back and accept it, or will you get involved and start making the rules?

Whether you like it or not, you're already in the game. You might as well learn how to play and win.

Reality Check: Facts Don't Win, Power Does

- Being right isn't enough. You can have all the evidence in the world, but if you don't have numbers or media pressure, it won't matter.
- Politicians don't care about logic; they care about pressure. They respond to threats to their professional image, their seat, and their funding.
- No one in power voluntarily gives up control. If change is going to happen, it has to be demanded and backed by real consequences for ignoring it.

Stop Whining, Start Winning

Corruption in healthcare and politics is real. It's frustrating, disheartening, and, if we're being honest, it makes you want to throw your hands up and walk away.

Here's the truth: **whining about corruption won't fix it**. Power concedes nothing unless forced.

You have two choices:

1. **Resuscitate Nursing**- Get the numbers to beat it. Organize. Mobilize. Outnumber your opposition.
2. **Keep going with the status quo**- That's exactly what they want. That's how they win.

I'm kidding, we both know number two isn't a viable option. So let's talk about how you Resuscitate Nursing.

We don't have time for fantasy. This book is about action. About reclaiming the soul of nursing before it's legislated, regulated, and mandated out of existence.

You can't fix what you don't name—and you sure can't win a war if you're still debating whether or not there's a fight.

Let's start there.

3
Identifying the Problem

"The symptoms of disease may be the same in two cases, but the conditions producing them may be different, and it is the conditions that must be altered."
- Florence Nightingale

Every movement begins with a spark. But don't romanticize it. That spark? It usually burns.

It burns with anger.
It burns with contempt.
It burns like acid eroding the esophagus of a patient with GERD.

It's that stinging deep down in your gut, knowing that something is wrong and *someone* has to do something about it.

The first step is naming what's broken and refusing to gaslight yourself into silence.

As with our patients, politics requires a good assessment of the problem. An appropriate assessment may take some time, but I promise it is worth it.

Everyone knows healthcare is "a mess," but what are the most compelling issues related to your job, network, hospital, or particular area?

Identifying the problem will benefit you by allowing for a comprehensive analysis, data gathering, identification of your enemies and allies, and so much more. You also want to pick the right fight at the right time. Choosing the right battle can provide you the opportunity to become known, respected, and effective.

On the other hand, choosing the wrong fight will result in demoralization, frustration, and even a loss of hope. Picking the wrong fight allows politicians to continue dominating the situation and reinforces the idea that it is futile to argue with them.

Picking the right fight at the wrong time can be equally detrimental, and you will want to avoid this.

First, start a list of pressing issues and ask what concerns other nurses have. What are the most pressing problems? Is it pay? Is it unrealistic expectations or added responsibilities? Are there policies that are failing or getting in the way?

What issues put a strain on nursing and patient safety? Are there moral dilemmas eroding nursing ethics? Do certain practices or protocols result in a loss of patient autonomy and informed decision making?

My guess is, if you're reading this book you've already identified a problem. However, you should do a little digging and ask those you work with what their opinions are about different issues and the potential solutions.

Once you have a list of problems and have narrowed them down to a couple of ideas, it is time to start refining them.

We know staffing is an issue, but simply going to leadership with the idea of "better staffing" is rather vague. It isn't likely to result in what you or your peers are looking for.

Why? Approaching in this manner is complaining, not demanding a solution. So what should you do? Again, our nursing practice prepares us for this, and we will use SMART goals to work on developing solutions.

SMART Goals

Grab the top 3-5 problems from your list and develop a SMART goal for them. You will want to gather a few other nurses and do this together. Keep things organized and use the worksheet found in the Resuscitating Nursing Workbook & Field manual or found on wtajourney.com/rnbook.

SMART goals help nurse advocates channel frustration into focused, effective action by providing a clear structure for change. SMART stands for:

- **S**pecific – Clear and focused
- **M**easurable – Can be tracked or counted
- **A**chievable – Realistic and within reach
- **R**elevant – Directly tied to your purpose
- **T**ime-bound – Has a deadline for completion

When advocating for change, especially in a system that often resists it, SMART goals give you the tools to act with precision and persistence. They help you build credibility, track wins, and maintain momentum. But we will add another letter to the acronym, creating "SMART-E" goals.

E will stand for Effect.

We always want to ask ourselves what the effect will be. We should consistently question ourselves, "Will this make meaningful change?"

Here are two examples of SMART-E goals:

Unsafe Nurse-to-Patient Ratios (Hospital-Level Goal)

SMART-E Goal:

By the end of the second quarter, the hospital will have hired at least 33% of the additional nursing positions required to meet evidence-based safe staffing ratios [or specific ratios you set based on evidence] on all inpatient units, with a progress report delivered to unit leadership and frontline staff at the end of the second quarter. This process will be repeated quarterly until staffing is maintained for one year.

- **Specific:** Targets hiring for safe nurse-to-patient ratios
- **Measurable:** Minimum benchmark set at 33% of required positions
- **Achievable:** One-third hiring/posting goal is a practical first phase
- **Relevant:** Improves patient safety, nurse retention, and organizational outcomes
- **Time-bound:** To be completed by the end of the second quarter, with transparent reporting
- **Effect:** Increases nurse availability at the bedside, reduces burnout, improves patient outcomes, and begins to rebuild trust between frontline staff and hospital leadership

Inadequate Orientation for New Nurses

SMART-E Goal:

Starting next month, all new nurses on orientation will be paired with preceptors who are assigned no more than four patients during the day shift and no more than five during the night shift for the first one-third of their scheduled floor orientation days. The education coordinator and unit leadership will review this adjustment monthly to assess the impact on patient outcomes and preceptor feedback.

- **Specific:** Limits preceptor assignments to ensure focused orientation and safe care
- **Measurable:** Applies to the first 1/3 of orientation days, with staffing caps clearly defined.
- **Achievable:** Targeted timeframe and staffing expectations make implementation feasible.
- **Relevant:** Supports both new nurse development and patient safety.
- **Time-bound:** Launches next month, with monthly reviews to guide continued implementation.
- **Effect:** Enhances new nurse confidence & trust of co-workers, reduces early turnover, improves patient safety, and supports long-term workforce stability by investing in effective mentorship, improves mentor satisfaction and drive to support professional and personal development of the new hire

These smart goals give us a frame of reference for hospital policies:

The hospital will maintain staffing ratios of _____. Currently, staffing ratios range between _____. Management must report the number of staff members needed for each unit to achieve its goal, and a minimum of ⅓ of the open positions must be posted.

Preceptors conducting the first ⅓ of new hire orientation must not have more than ___ patients [list out different units if needed]. If appropriate staffing is unavailable, management will provide assistance on the floor until the proper ratios are established.

When building out the goals, you must always ask yourself:

Will this make a meaningful change?

Or, is this kicking the can down the road?

All too often, nurses are offered short-term solutions or excuses with no fundamental changes. If you are taking up these fights, the last thing you want to do is invest your time and energy into something that fails to improve the long-term situation.

If you are working on SMART-E goals, the chances of making real change are enhanced, because you present precisely what you want or expect with a measurable outcome. Measurable outcomes provide a point for accountability for politicians, and evaluating the effect helps you remain accountable to your mission.

Negotiations

This is important- know precisely what you want, be clear about the parameters, and accept nothing less.

Do not compromise on the necessities.

Don't get me wrong, this isn't about being belligerent. It isn't about disrespect or refusing to discuss the issues. You must remember that politicians, including management, will try to squeak by with the BARE minimum.

Let's be honest, when we think about how our advocacy efforts have gone in the past, we can see how politicians are typically great manipulators- I mean, negotiators. We will discuss this further in Chapter Six, Strategic Communication.

I want to be clear, though, this isn't a negotiation that you are demanding for something unrealistic, like a 3:1 ratio on med-surg units.

Sometimes when we think about negotiating, it is confused with haggling. We imagine starting with absolute extremes, nearing the unreasonable space, and working our way to the middle. We don't want to demand something unnecessary, which is why we can say, no compromises. There may be aspects of your goal that may be negotiable; it is up to you to decide on those beforehand.

Are you willing to allow the plan to be implemented over a year instead of nine months?

Sadly, in many instances in nursing, the bare minimum will likely seem extreme because healthcare standards have been eroded. It is vital in times when the politicians are trying to make you feel unreasonable or as though you are "extreme", that you remember- **the extremes define the middle.**

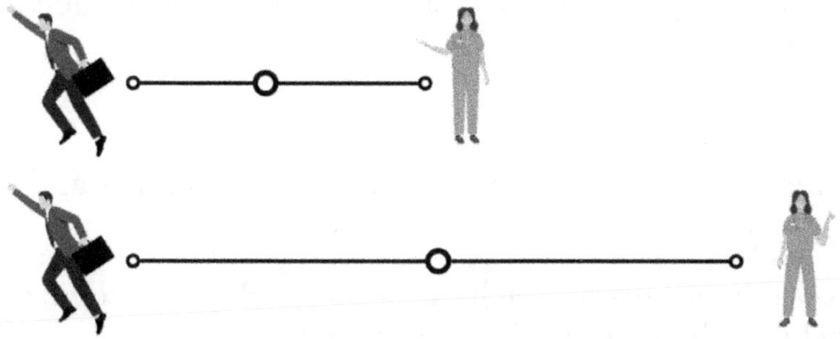

> ***Pro Tip:*** The idea of extremes defining the middle comes from a concept called the "Overton Window." Essentially, the concept means politicians will stick to a "safe" comfort zone consisting of what is deemed acceptable by corporate leadership, and rarely, the public. It is "safe" because it is a "moderate" stance. When competing ideas are presented with a wider threshold for what is acceptable, this redefines the Overton window or the "middles."

So, while our requests are not actually extreme, they just feel extreme to a broken system, we must maintain that strong stance for exactly what we want.

Let's look at this in a practical way.

If I draw a line with an anchor point on the left side of the page extending two inches to the right, the middle hits at one inch. Then, if I use the same anchor point on the left side of the page and draw a four-inch line, the middle shifts out farther, to two inches.

The middle point of each of these lines are drastically different. Now let's apply the politician's preference, or the issue's current status, to the left anchor point. This might also be referenced as the "status quo". We know these politicians want to stay in this "safe" space, and they will do everything in their power to keep it that way. They know what they want, to protect corporate interests, and they are not going to budge unless they are forced.

The demands made by nursing agents of change are the endpoint to the right. This is the endpoint you have control over. If these two lines measure progress and change, which endpoint do you want to set?

The one at one inch or the one at four inches?

Which endpoint, or demand, will maximize your efforts and ensure appropriate safety and patient care?

While we will work towards achieving our goals, we recognize that it will likely not happen on the first attempt.

We know that there will be negotiations and debate. There will be excuses and whining. We have a better chance at getting what is needed for change if we demand what we want and settle for nothing less.

When progress is made, you will continue to "double down" efforts to achieve your initial goal.

I am belaboring this point for a reason. Many will argue for incrementalism. Incrementalism involves planning to return and take small bites out of a problem, thereby increasing tolerance for the solution over time. This kind of tactic works wonders for lobbyists and those with money and time to burn.

Patients and nurses do not have time or money to burn.

We cannot play the political game of incrementalism.

Your requests should be firmly founded in patient safety and ethical principles. Starting with precisely what you want and not beyond that gives you credibility. This eliminates any real argument against what you are demanding and shifts the politicians into a situation where they are simply whining.

EXPOSE THAT.

Sometimes, it may *feel* like they have legitimate excuses for not giving you exactly what you want. They will inevitably throw loads of "reasons" at you, but when you build your foundation on realistic expectations, it is much easier to rebuke them.

Use the "E-Effect" of your SMART-E goal to recenter and regroup if your army begins to be swayed. **This will give you the power to use the common-sense approach as both a shield and a weapon.**

Sometimes, when working through complex issues, intermediate goals may be necessary. Like mile markers on a road trip, these goals show progress and help change makers recognize progress, create motivation, and prevent demoralization. The key difference between compromise and creating intermediate or short-term goals depends on your words and how you frame these situations to politicians and other change makers. Words matter.

We will talk more about this in Chapter Six, Strategic Communication, but for now, remember to acknowledge the progress and always point back to the ultimate goal and what needs to be done to get there.

"Posting an open position is a great first step; however, patient safety and nursing satisfaction will suffer until we have trained nurses at the bedside. We expect…"

When you present what you are demanding, you can also intertwine the expectation of further action on intermediate goals. Considering the staffing goal above, it would be unreasonable to expect all positions to be filled within one quarter. Setting the expectation at 33% will result in a measurable change without creating undesired consequences, such as a lack of preceptors. However, the last line, stating that the process will continue each quarter until staffing numbers are obtained, sets the expectation for continued action.

The goals outlined above are rough examples and must be tailored to your area of focus. They will require a bit of investigation and documentation, which I will refer to as "receipts".

When attacking a problem, planning will be key. Grab the necessary information, or receipts, to support your claims. Obtain documentation that shows the issue, which may include copies of staffing grids and unit schedules to illustrate the gaps. It may be interviews, commentary from new nurses and their preceptors, or patient experiences.

Depending on state recording laws, recording conversations or meetings may be helpful. It is imperative that you know state laws regarding recordings and contact an attorney with any questions. There are many times when I wish I had "worn a wire" and caught just how critical staffing was at an old employer. The conversations during staffing huddles were intense and terrifying. I left those meetings with a pit in my stomach because I knew patients were at risk and there was no "good" answer.

> ***Pro Tip:*** Double-check with an attorney about your state recording laws and their implications. Recordinglaw.com is one of many resources you can use to educate yourself and understand the topic a bit more.

Any problem that presents will have some form of a receipt that you can use to show the problem. This information will also help push the political pain points of politicians. I can't stress this next point enough.

Nothing a nurse does should put a patient or their privacy at risk.

As you collect your receipts, be sure to protect patient privacy. Your receipts must be stored securely and in a place you can access, even if you quit or lose your job. They are not good to you if you can't get to them.

If persecuted or fired for your efforts, keeping ethical and accurate documentation may be the difference between losing your job and license. For some whistle-blowers, following these principles has made all the difference.

Finally, the last tip for identifying the problem is to narrow down who is responsible for the solution. We will face unit-wide, institutional, industry, or state-level problems. Digging into the issue and identifying who has the authority over the problem, and if any institutional, state, or federal policies or regulations dictate how the problem is created or solved.

Consider the chain of command and follow the steps when possible. Sometimes, you bypass the hospital and go straight to the state legislature, but problems can often be solved at the institutional level. This is excellent news because, as you learned, politics is a numbers game. You have direct access and sometimes a connection with many nurses in your institution.

In contrast, you may be disconnected entirely from the nurses across your state simply because of the sheer number or distance. Effectively mobilizing fewer people is typically easier than thousands or hundreds of thousands.

Another critical aspect of knowing who is responsible for the solution to your problem is that you can effectively and appropriately mobilize your team. If you fail to identify the correct politician and mobilize your team against an individual who is incapable of making change, you and your team will have wasted time and resources. The risk is that you will likely become frustrated and feel the fight isn't worth it. Guard your time and team from these kinds of mistakes.

Knowing the responsible party, tracing the steps, and showing the process can also help protect you and your team from politicians who would rather deflect and falsely claim their hands are tied, hiding behind legalities that don't apply. In these instances, have them provide the receipts. They are not exempt. Hold them accountable for the claims they make.

We will close it out with one final note on this section. As a nurse, you not only have the moral and ethical responsibility to report unsafe conditions, but you also have the legal responsibility.

When I worked in the hospitals, the nurses were devastated; we did our best to serve our patients and encourage each other. Poor staffing and inexperienced nurses were the impetus of sentinel events.

This time was a crucial turning point in my career. I was a nurse for 3-4 years, night shift charge nurse on a 24-bed telemetry unit with three new nurses. I started that shift praying that everyone would make it out alive…

I was sitting at the charge desk, working on a new admit in the era before physicians entered their own electronic orders.

I remember it all so clearly. I was hustling and trying to get the chart ready for the nurse so I could get back to my patients as well. I was deeply focused when I heard a strange noise.

I looked up from the desk and realized the door to the room across from me was shut. From the charge report, I knew the patient in that room was restrained, confused, and getting tube feeds. I leapt up and ran into the room. I found this elderly, confused, restrained patient choking on his tube feeding because the bed was flat.

This was not my patient, but I knew he was a full code. I yelled out for help and slapped the code button. Mind you, there were five staff members in the unit, including me. I stopped the tube feed, removed the restraints, and rolled the patient onto his side.

I searched for suction tubing and couldn't find any. Luckily, the one tech on the floor hit the door at that moment. He was able to call a rapid response overhead while running for suction. He also called the patient's nurse, but she didn't arrive until after respiratory care had arrived and we had suctioned, and the patient completely crashed.

We ended up doing CPR on that patient, and I will never forget the way the tube feed bubbled out of him. It was evident to us that the tube feed was not coming from the stomach. The patient's emaciated abdomen was sunken in, and the gurgling was a tell-tale sign.

In those moments, despite working to save this man's life, the guilt had already crept in. The sorrow over the whole situation saturated everyone in the room. But the most disturbing thing is how wretched his final HOURS on earth must have been. God bless him.

I also felt terrible for his nurse. I knew she would carry this with her the rest of her life. I am not sure that I ever knew what led to the situation.

Did she leave the head of the bed down?

Were his restraints in the proper position so that he could have lowered the head of the bed?

Who shut the door? Was it intentional? Would it have mattered?

I don't know if those questions were ever asked. I don't know that it would have changed anything. Sadly, at the beginning of that shift, the outgoing charge and I discussed how the staffing situation was primed for a disaster like this. It was the status quo.

Our new hires were recent graduates with no experience, and were oriented in a rush with heavy patient loads, both in terms of volume and acuity.

Nurses on our unit made reports as appropriate within the institution and pushed for better staffing because this was not an isolated incident. Sentinel events happened regularly.

Our management knew the issues, the whole hospital knew how bad things were on our unit and a couple of others, yet nothing changed.

When nothing changed at the hospital level, many of us reported to the Joint Commission on Accreditation. We naively thought this accrediting/auditing body would take action and help us protect our patients.

We were so very wrong.

Investigations were done, and we were told that the hospital put procedures in place to protect patients, but nothing changed. We felt as if there was nothing more that could have been done.

We were left hopeless and abandoned. Turnover continued to accelerate, and we became more distrustful of the administration and the industry overall. The nurses gave up trying to make a change. Instead, they did one of three things: double down on personal accountability, exit the system, or accept that failure was inevitable.

I doubled down with personal responsibility in an impossible situation. Taking the weight of this burden led to moral injury and my eventual exit from bedside nursing. Those who didn't double down seemed to have accepted that these situations happen and that it was just a part of hospital nursing. They accepted defeat and resigned themselves to remaining in "tele-hell," a moniker used both as a badge of courage and despair. To this day, over a decade later, things have not improved. I hear things are worse than ever.

> ***Pro Tip:*** Moral distress and injury are often mislabeled as burnout and are a significant cause of nursing attrition. To overcome moral injury, you must live in congruence with your beliefs. By resuscitating nursing, that is exactly what you are doing. Learn more about moral injury a wajourney.com/mip.

A couple of years ago, I was reading through Indiana's nurse practice act, which mostly consisted of a short portion of state code guiding the procedure for nursing licensure, and I found something that shook me to the core.

Indiana nurses are instructed in Indiana state law to "report any unprofessional conduct which may jeopardize the patient/client safety" to the attorney general's office. In our state, the Attorney General has authority over all professional licenses, including oversight of licensed healthcare facilities. Looking back, I wonder how different our complaints would have landed had we made reports to the licensing board, through the Attorney General, instead of an accrediting body like the Joint Commission.

That distinction matters.

Accrediting bodies, such as the Joint Commission, are independent, private organizations that evaluate hospitals based on quality measures and performance benchmarks. Their focus is more about improvement than enforcement; while influential, accreditation is voluntary.

Whereas a licensing board is part of the state government and exists to enforce the minimum legal and safety standards that facilities must meet to operate. This includes aspects such as sanitation, staffing, infection control, and patient protection. Accountability to the licensing board isn't optional if a facility wants to stay open.

The Attorney General has the legal authority to investigate, discipline, and even shut down facilities that fail to meet state requirements. When patient safety is at risk, legal enforcement carries more weight than mere suggestions made by accrediting agencies to improve.

We will never know if those situations would have been remedied if we had reported to the Attorney General. However, I pray that empowering those still at the bedside with this information will help create that change.

This is a perfect example of the importance of knowing the chain of command and who is responsible for change. At the time, we thought we were doing the right thing. We thought the Joint Commission would help us protect our patients- that is what we were led to believe.

Now I can't help but wonder if that was by design, an intentional deception as a layer of protection for hospitals.

That is a problem for another day.

Once you've named the problems and know who is responsible for fixing them, you can't unsee them; no more illusions. No more pretending the house isn't on fire. You're responsible for triage. Just like you can't be in every patient room at once, you can't take on every fight at once.

Your patient is our profession, and the disease is multisystem failure. Your treatment plan must be strategic because it's time to stop documenting harm and start delivering change.

Now let's talk about how to pick your first battle.

4
Prioritizing the Best Battle

"Unless we are making progress in our nursing every year, every month, every week, take my word for it, we are going back."
- Florence Nightingale

When a patient is in multisystem failure, we don't just throw the kitchen sink at them and hope for the best. We stabilize what's critical first. We prioritize. We intervene where it matters most.

Our profession isn't much different. Issues range from minor policy changes to larger issues like nursing retention and the abject failure of the system to protect patients. In the last step, you identified topics specific to your area of focus. You learned about them, built smart goals, and gathered "receipts."

As a nurse, you are a fixer, so you must fight the urge to fix all the problems simultaneously. Looking at the sheer amount of work in front of you may make you feel like walking away.

You won't.
You are a change-maker.
You are dedicated, strong, and intelligent.
You are a powerful force to be reckoned with.

Don't forget that!

You are a powerful force to be reckoned with.

I say this with all the love in the world, although you are likely a stellar multitasker- fighting all the issues at once is NOT a way you can effectively make change.

You will undoubtedly need to continue to remind yourself that many battles are worth fighting, but not all are worth fighting *now*.

Some battles will be prioritized over others out of necessity. Still, most should be sought with surgical precision, honing in on the isolated area and carefully dissecting the source of concern.

You must remember that you aren't walking away from problems; you're choosing to fight with surgical precision, not recklessly or haphazardly.

Why Picking the Right Battle Matters

To be truly effective, you cannot split your time and talent. You are already engaged in many different activities. From regular working hours, committees, family, volunteering, and hobbies. Your time is limited. You deserve some balance. The people you lead depend on you to make wise decisions.

For many people, the idea of being a change-maker is appealing, but the amount of time and energy required is daunting and often leads to walking away before the goal is achieved, or even getting off the ground.

When you pick the right battle, you can channel your limited time and energy into a specific area with a greater chance of success. Your messaging becomes clear and concise while stirring up action in those around you. Effective communication of the problem *and plan* fuels growth. Efforts are amplified by those prepared to get behind your cause and even help lead the charge.

As we discussed, people want to be effective at making change, so picking the right battle at the right time is crucial to building a track record of success and avoiding burnout.

Obviously, picking the right battle will advance nursing professionalism, patient safety, ethical practices, and nursing satisfaction.

But how do you know?

When the world (of nursing) is on fire, it may seem like a good idea to start dumping water on everything, but we know that is ineffective. With limited water (i.e., resources or time), you will quickly run out. How do you prioritize a specific area over another when the crises seem to be at every turn?

If you are going to be an effective change-maker, you will have to learn how to discern which fights are hot, which fights are not, and how to avoid the distractions thrown like hand grenades designed to jolt you off your game.

The moment you show promise of being a change maker, all kinds of people will toss you grenades in the form of ideas. The politicians in your life are exceptionally good at this.

Their goal is to overwhelm you, talk you out of continuing, and create dissent among you and your peers. They want you to go away, and they will do anything to help that process along. We will discuss this further later.

Some of the ideas presented will be worthy causes, but may not significantly impact your problems. They may be caused by challenges in other areas of your setting, generalized industry issues, or problems found by well-meaning peers who see you as the "go-to" person.

When new ideas are presented, you need to triage them.

Don't just jump into action based on emotion, anxiety, or a knee-jerk reaction. You must ask yourself, "Do I have to fight this battle right now?"

To know that, you must identify the type of battle it is. In the heat of the moment, nearly all battles feel like life or death.

One of the most valuable lessons I learned from that political seminar was that three types of battles exist.

1. *Survival*
2. *Obligatory*
3. *Opportunity*

When I first heard this, I laughed. There is no way that all the political battles will fall into these three categories.

The longer I have been an active agent of change, the more true I have found it to be. For the most part, these categories are self-explanatory, but let's do a quick review.

1. **Survival battles** are the ones in which you are literally going to die, politically or professionally. These battles are direct, severe attacks on you or your organization. They will end your career or position at a particular facility.

   These battles are going to be few and far between. They are actually pretty rare. It is easy to want to label the fights we face as "survival." This creates a sense of urgency, *but these urges are driven by emotion and not reality.*

2. **Obligatory battles** are the fights you get dragged into, not because someone brought the idea to you, but because it started elsewhere, and if you don't join in, problems will arise. These problems may include losing standing as the expert, creating a wedge in the group you are working with, or even causing your group to fracture.

It was described to me that your younger sibling picked a fight, and now you have no choice but to help out or face trouble at home. In the past 5 years, I have only had 1-2 of these fights, and they usually eliminate themselves.

3. **Opportunity battles** are the most common. Your "life" is not in jeopardy, and it is optional with the potential to grow your cause. These are abundant and therefore require careful consideration to ensure the best use of your resources.

Again, the most abundant type of fight will be an opportunity battle, not survival or obligatory. It is tempting to think that all battles are do-or-die, and that is why we need a tool to help us objectify some of these highly charged ideas, or even just FOMO, the fear of missing out. I know that seems funny, but I promise there will be issues that crop up, and you will be tempted to deviate from your plan because a shiny new object appears.

There will be times when "friends" come to tell you about a big problem. There will be times when you are getting close to an accomplishment, and your political foes will try to give you whiplash. In any of these situations, doing a risk-benefit analysis will help you triage what steps to take next.

We will use a Strategic Triage Framework to turn subjective issues into more objective assessments. The process is like a risk-benefit analysis, looking at the risks, benefits, alternatives, and pros and cons of each.

Strategic Triage Framework

The Process

To complete a Strategic Triage Framework (STF), you will work through a series of scored questions with key team members. Working with a team on the STF will be essential to the process. Discussions, diverse ideas, and varied perspectives ensure a more robust conversation and sometimes a debate. This is a healthy response.

As the leader, you must ensure that things remain civil. Suppose you find that you have a team member who tries to bully the others into submission or turns everything into a philosophical debate. In that case, it is perfectly acceptable to stop inviting them to work on the STF.

When working in a group, it will be imperative to document your findings. Not just the score, but the key points of conversation. Just like with nursing interventions, you must write down your rationale and the number ratings. The only thing worse than skipping documentation is not doing the STF in the first place.

Writing down reasons that you think are obvious is still essential, as over time, these may slip your mind. You will keep the completed STF in a folder to reference it. There are multiple helpful worksheets in the Resuscitating Nursing Workbook and Field Manual, some of which are found on wtajourney.com/rnbook.

There are two main reasons for reviewing the STF. First, to evaluate the battle once it is over, and second, to assess if a new fight should be taken up. As nurses, we are used to doing evaluations. It is a natural habit for us because it is ingrained in us to evaluate the effectiveness of interventions for our patients.

Nurses are naturals when it comes to process improvement because assessing the changes in our patients is imperative. So, evaluating the accuracy of your STF at the end of a fight should come as second nature.

Review your work, make notes of unexpected deviations or areas you didn't anticipate, and grow along the way, refining your skills.

The other instance for review would be when a new battle is presented and appears to take precedence. If a new idea surfaces, it's not a battle of survival, and your team begins talking about changing gears, you can complete the STF on the new idea and compare. This can be invaluable in redirecting energy that could otherwise be wasted or create division.

You must remember that the STF assesses the individual fight. The comparison happens ***after*** the STF is completed for each issue separately, not within the framework. Everyone on the team has the responsibility to remind each other of this. When conducting an STF, you assess the fight solely based on that fight's merits. You are not taking into account any other factors or battles. After you evaluate the fight's merits, you can pull one or more other STFs together and compare the fights more objectively.

You may find it helpful to review your STF periodically during a fight, or if you are struggling to continue pushing, become frustrated, stray off track, circumstances change, or feel like things aren't going well. The STF may inspire you along the journey and remind you why you are doing things the way you are. It can also help redirect your actions.

Basic Rules

Don't triage alone.
Whenever possible, complete the framework with trusted allies or team members. Others may see blind spots or offer clarity you can't see alone.

Write it down. Always.
Record your scores and the rationale for each one. This allows for reflection later, prevents emotional reactivity, and reveals patterns over time.

Each issue gets scored on its merit.
No comparing battles during scoring. Avoid ranking or pitting problems against each other while completing the form.

10s are rarities.
It is tempting to rate all things as 10s, but this is simply not reality. You will seldom have a score of 10 on individual questions. Use them sparingly.

Compare after all are scored.
Once multiple issues are scored, compare the final numbers to determine priority. But not before! This protects objectivity.

Focus on one main issue at a time.
The framework is not for multitasking advocacy. Use it to laser in on where your energy can have the most strategic impact. If your group or organization grows and you can delegate, you may strategically decide to expand.

Trust the score.
Even if an issue feels emotionally important, if the triage score is low, it may not be worth your limited energy right now.

Revisit as conditions change or after victory.
This is not a one-and-done tool. If the political winds shift, circumstances escalate, or you find renewed energy, re-score.

The Questions

Let's dive in.

First, I am going to list all the questions for the Strategic Triage Framework, then we will go through each of them in more detail.

What kind of battle is this?

If it is anything except a survival battle, ask:
Will this detract from the efforts I am currently carrying out?

Score the following questions from -10 to +10:

1. Win or lose, will this action attract more nurses, patients, or financial support to our advocacy efforts?
2. Win or lose, will this strengthen allies, advocates, or organizations working toward similar goals?
3. Win or lose, will this weaken or expose the institutions or individuals responsible for unethical or unsafe practices, ie, political enemies?
4. Split Decision: Only one of these will be scored.

   a. If we lose, how much ground will be lost in terms of nurse autonomy or patient rights?

   b. If we win, how much will this improve nurse autonomy or patient rights?

5. What is the hassle factor, time, risk, emotional drain, or backlash involved in taking this action?

Let's go ahead and review the purpose of each part of the STF.

What Kind of Battle is This?

Remember, there are three types of battles: survival, obligatory, and opportunity. Your team will evaluate objectively which kind of battle this particular fight is.

Being deliberate about this will help you avoid knee-jerk reactions. Then, if the fight is anything other than a survival battle, you will consider: *"Is this a distraction from our current mission?" "How could that be used against you?"*

Remember: Put your team's thoughts in writing.

You can always come back and review if you or one of your team members starts to feel the urgency has shifted. Do a recap with the members of your team and stay objective.

Score the following questions from -10 to +10:

> *Win or lose, will this action attract more nurses, patients, or financial support to our advocacy efforts?*

Just for fighting this battle, win or lose- this is key. You are not focusing on one outcome or the other. You are looking at both and determining if simply bringing light to the issue will unite people around it, if they will take action, and if they will donate towards advocacy. List the kinds of people this will bring in: nurses, patients, and certain types of each. Will doctors or other staff members join in? What parts of this fight will activate others?

If you take up this battle, the information in this section can and will help you plan who to engage with, what talking points to use, and make planning more efficient.

> *Win or lose, will this strengthen allies, advocates, or organizations working toward similar goals?*

Allies come in different forms. They can be other organizations, peer groups, other professions, middle management, friendly politicians, etc. List your known allies and consider any new allies that this fight might bring to the table.

Why is it important to consider how picking this fight will help or harm your allies? Simple, you don't want friendly fire in war; politics, or on the battlefield. To put it in nursing terms, it is kind of like balancing treatments for a renal patient in acute heart failure. Before taking action, we have to be prepared for how causing harm to our allies could be detrimental to our cause and long-term viability.

Conversely, if fighting a battle, again win or lose, will help our allies, this can be a huge boost not only in our organization but in those who work similarly or in parallel to us. Choosing fights that will help, or at least be inconsequential for our allies, comes with significant benefits.

If it will rally the ally into joining the fight, we strengthen and build our case, creating "crossfire" where the politician is now facing pushback from more than one group. Developing crossfire is incredibly beneficial in nailing down your political foes.

If the fight is negligible and our allies can continue doing their own thing, we don't develop a benefit from it; however, this is much preferred over burdening our allies. If the chosen battle is seen as an obligatory fight by an ally, they may be irritated because it costs them time and resources to join in.

However, avoiding fights that harm our allies is preferable if possible. If your allies are hurt, it may cause discord, internal arguments, and a lack of trust. More time could be spent fighting with friends rather than the common foe. This is imperative to avoid. In some cases, this may be unavoidable or show signs of shifting allegiances. Be sure to evaluate any fight that can cause harm to allies carefully.

Win or lose, will this weaken or expose the institutions or individuals responsible for unethical or unsafe practices, ie, political enemies?

Again, list your potential "enemies" who seek to promote unethical or unsafe practices. You will want to consider what groups, individuals, and political leaders could stand in opposition to your efforts. These "enemies" are not always easy to spot. Just like with your allies, you want to list the possibilities and consider them carefully.

Don't hesitate to add new "enemies" to the list when you find them; this may help you in the future. Evaluating your enemies up front will help steer planning once you decide on a particular fight.

After all, going into battle, your ultimate goal is to create enough pressure to make a change. People and corporations only make change when it is easy or they can no longer stand the pressure for not doing the right thing.

In your notes, you want to be able to pinpoint the pain points of your enemies and understand how this fight will impact them.

An important point to consider is if fighting this fight will BENEFIT your ally. If your enemies can fundraise or list build by opposing you, this would be represented as a negative number. Don't miss the fact that picking certain fights may bolster your political foe through people or money. Be sure to take these into account.

Split Decision

The other questions have deliberately focused on fighting the fight, not the outcome. This is where we shift gears. In this question, we specifically address the outcome. Only one of these two questions will be scored. It was challenging to wrap my mind around how to answer only one.

What wasn't explained to me is that, when picking **battles of survival**, you will answer question A, or "the cost to the cause," if the battle is lost. This is because if you win a battle of survival, you are likely not improving your conditions; you are simply maintaining what was before.

If you win, you live to fight another day. If you lose, you are no longer a player in the game.

In **battles of opportunity**, you almost certainly will answer question B: how much will this improve our cause? If you lose a battle of opportunity, you are simply remaining status quo, so there is no actual "loss." It just means you revise your plan and keep fighting. However, if you win, you want to know how far this moves the needle.

Are your efforts going to be worth the fight? This can sometimes make or break a fight. Be realistic on this question because it can substantially change your final outcome. **Obligatory battles** are often going to fall into this category as well.

a. *If we lose, how much ground will be lost in terms of nurse autonomy or patient rights?*

For this question, think about all the possible outcomes: job loss, frustration, decreased patient care, patient injury or death, increased patient ratios, loss of a dedicated charge nurse. These areas are all potentially seen as battles of survival.

<u>The more egregious the policy or stipulation, the more the number will INCREASE.</u>

This feels backwards. I get it. Assigning something "negative" a positive number does not feel right. But remember, the "higher" the total score, the stronger the rationale for the fight is. So when you answer the COST, the greater the HARM, the HIGHER the number.

So, if there is a wild policy stating that staffing ratios may be 6:1 in the ICU, this would be rated a 10. A positive 10. 6:1 in an ICU would result in the loss of all the nurses, and patients would certainly die due to improper oversight and care. It's plain and simple. This would be all hands on deck, do or die, pull out all the stops kind of fight.

b. *If we win, how much will this improve nurse autonomy or patient rights?*

Again, review your outcomes. In this case, winning is a battle of opportunity; if you lose, you don't actually lose anything because you're staying at the status quo. However, the level of victory can vary greatly.

For example, let's say that an obligatory battle was started for a "unit-based shared-governance council." This battle is not improving things; it gives unit nurses a "seat at the table" or a "chance to be heard."

While this isn't a bad thing, it certainly isn't going to directly move the needle on patient safety or change any actual policy or practice. It will add to the nurses' responsibilities, and there is no guarantee that the "voices" will be taken into account or provide meaningful change to the policies enacted by the administration.

My number will be relatively low in answering the question of how much this will improve nurse autonomy or patient rights. Perhaps a two or a three. It won't be negative, but again, minimal direct positive impact, and the true issues are kicked down the road rather than being addressed.

However, the rating would be pretty high if a fight arises regarding strict statewide staffing grids with reasonable maximums, and the requirement for management to work the floor should staffing not be available. I would probably assign a rating of seven or eight.

This is a significant win and would ensure safe staffing *and* an incentive for management to ensure appropriate staffing.

I hope those examples give you a good picture of how to answer the question. The greater the win, the greater the number. It is more intuitive than the other.

The Hassle Factor

What is the hassle factor: time, risk, emotional drain, or backlash, involved in taking this action?

The final question: What is the hassle factor? This question makes things interesting, and you may or may not choose to include it in your final score. It can be looked at independently or lumped in. There are times when a low-hassle fight will pop up amid a larger fight and may be worth fighting.

However, that means the fight must move the needle and be incredibly low on the hassle factor. However, if you are adding this score into your overall rating, you have to remember this score will be INVERSE. **The lower the hassle, the HIGHER the score.**

So, if a fight arises during a bigger battle but takes little to no work and can pay off, it is likely that I would jump into that fight. However, the low hassle factor means minimal time investment, both in duration and intensity. Meaning I might invest 30-60 minutes, and the results will be achieved in 3 days. It makes the fight a no-brainer, especially if the benefit to patients, nurses, or healthcare is significant.

However, looking at long-term battles, the Hassle Factor can still help determine the overall score or compare multiple battles with similar scores on the other portions of the STF.

Once you have completed each question, add the scores and follow the process for the other fights. Once you have completed the STF for each fight, you can compare them based on their merits.

You may not always choose the highest-scoring fight; however, using the Strategic Triage Framework will help you understand the complexities of the fights and will help you prioritize and plan your battles as you get started.

You are standing at the starting line of real, meaningful change.

You don't need a fancy title or an official leadership role to make an impact. You only need clarity, purpose, and a little strategy. Choosing your battles wisely through the Strategic Triage Framework isn't about backing down from a fight. It's about preserving strength, maximizing impact, and building lasting movement.

You won't fix everything at once, and that's precisely why you'll succeed.

You will fix the *right* thing, at the *right* time, in the *right* way.

Through each strategic action you take, you will inspire others to step forward, speak up, and join you.

Change is contagious.

Leadership is contagious.

And you, nurse, are precisely the kind of contagiousness our profession needs.

Using the Strategic Triage Framework does more than make your work manageable. It protects you. It shields you from the fear of missing out when a dozen worthy causes call your name. It arms you against distractions thrown by leaders, politicians, even your own team members, or the daily chaos of the news cycle. By focusing on one strong, clear issue at a time, you preserve your momentum and your sanity while making it much harder for opponents to undermine you.

Choosing a single, public-facing battle makes it exponentially harder for politicians to divide and conquer your team. It reduces their ability to twist your words, stall by "agreeing in principle," or quietly gutting your efforts while smiling to your face. When you stay laser-focused, their political maneuvering becomes obvious to you *and* to the people you mobilize. Your laser focus makes it harder for them to confuse your base, and easier for you to expose their games.

Understand this: politicians thrive on disorganization and vague frustration.

They love it when advocates show up mad but messy. Broad issues like "the healthcare system is broken" let them nod sympathetically, promise to "look into it," and stall for years. But when you show up with sharp, specific demands, like amending a section of policy or changing a staffing ratio, you corner them. You force action or expose their unwillingness to act.

> ***Pro Tip:*** If you are unsure about what unwillingness to act looks like, revisit chapter four's section "Knowing when you have pushed the right Button."

Focus isn't just a strategy. It's a survival skill. It keeps your team unified, prevents personality clashes from becoming fatal distractions, and ensures your energy builds over time instead of fizzling out. It protects you from being baited into small, meaningless "wins" that dilute your mission. It gives you the power to stand firm, to drive real change, and to keep moving even when the forces against you would prefer you wandering lost in a thousand different directions.

The road ahead will not always be smooth, but it will be worth it. Now that you understand how to pick battles, have a way to objectify them, and are getting geared up for battle, you need to learn about building your team…

Level Up Your Leadership

Don't just read about the Strategic Triage Framework, use it. Grab a notebook or a trusted colleague and triage one issue today. Strategic leadership isn't about doing everything; it's about doing the right thing, right now.

5
Building Your Team

"Let whoever is in charge keep this simple question in her head—(not, how can I always do this right thing myself?)—but how can I provide for this right thing to be always done?"

- Florence Nightingale

Your excitement is building, and you've probably already told a friend or two about this book and your plans for change. Some are receptive and maybe even excited, but I'll bet others are disparaging or discouraging.

It's OK. That's normal.

Remember our earlier discussion: don't waste precious energy trying to convince those who disagree or aren't interested.

Focus on those who lean in.

Focus on those who get that spark in their eye.

Follow up with *them*.

Keep sharing information, but don't fall into the trap of *only* sharing information.

When someone shows excitement, they aren't just looking for inspiration. They're signaling that they are ready for action. Tap into that. They aren't just encouragement, they *are* resources, potential team members, and volunteers.

Trust me, you cannot do this alone.

Starting a movement can feel overwhelming. This will differ even if you've led projects inside the traditional system. You won't have the built-in structure or resources you're used to.

You are the system now.

Necessary Roles

You are responsible for keeping the wheels on the wagon and keeping it moving.

You must know the roles to delegate to be an effective leader and build a functional team. These aren't about titles; they're about function. Pay close attention to the people who show up; you'll start to spot their natural skills and talents.

Here are the critical roles you'll want to identify:

- **The Front-Facing Advocate** becomes the public voice of the movement, the one who speaks at meetings, talks to the media, energizes the base, and becomes the rallying point when momentum slows.
- **The Strategist** thinks several moves ahead. They help the team stay sharp, avoid obvious traps, and position efforts for the maximum political and cultural impact.
- **The Organizer** keeps the wheels turning behind the scenes. They ensure meetings happen, tasks get assigned, lists are maintained, contacts updated, and no good idea falls through the cracks just because life gets busy.

- **The Communicator** crafts the message. They build the talking points, create handouts, draft social media posts, and ensure that everything the team says is sharp, clear, and consistent.
- **The Researcher** digs deep for facts, data, policies, and real-world examples. They ensure your movement isn't just emotional but backed by hard evidence and defensible points.
- **The Sharer** takes the message directly to the people. They are the connectors, educators, and grassroots champions who tell their friends, network at events, and help the message spread like wildfire.

In addition to these, there are a few **bonus roles** that can supercharge your movement if you can find them:

- **The Recon Scout** quietly monitors political developments, media stories, and internal opposition. They bring early warnings about opportunities or sabotage, so your team can stay one step ahead.
- **The Relationship Builder** focuses on strategic alliances. They build bridges to other nurses, patient groups, civic leaders, or even sympathetic insiders who can strengthen your influence.
- **The Logistics Captain** handles the behind-the-scenes mechanics: booking rooms, printing flyers, and setting up event tables. They are the quiet powerhouse that keeps events and actions running smoothly.
- **The Mentor** (even if unofficial) offers emotional support, wisdom, and a long view. When the fight gets hard, and it will, you'll need someone who can remind you why the work matters and that persistence pays off.

That may seem overwhelming, thinking about finding people to fill all those roles, but don't worry, it will happen organically as long as you're paying attention.

Let's dig a little deeper into the different roles.

The First Three Roles

The Front-Facing Advocate, Strategist, and Organizer will ultimately be your responsibility until you have a few battle-tested colleagues. I'm going to say that again: **battle-tested colleagues**, people who have not only read this book but who have run the ropes with you.

Until you build a high level of trust with key people, everything will be run by you before being released. That doesn't mean micromanaging, but you must ensure a consistent message that aligns with your goals.

Taking a no-nonsense approach to politics is not easy. It is not for the faint of heart. Many people, especially nurses, are drawn in by the hope of diplomacy. They want access. They want a seat at the table. And often, they think that's where the real change happens.

The illusion of change occurring simply by having a seat at the table is one of the oldest tricks in the book. And if you aren't careful, that illusion will infiltrate your team and rot it from the inside out. You and your growing movement can't afford that kind of sabotage. I've seen it happen more than once and nearly been a victim myself.

The only reason I wasn't taken down was because I used **layers of trust**. I didn't just hand someone a role because they showed up once or said the right thing. I watched. I tested. I paid attention to how they handled pressure, criticism, and disappointment.

I gave small tasks first and observed how they were handled.

Did the individual follow through?

Did they stay strong when things got hard?

It is easy to fall victim to the deception of politicians when the stakes are high. If your colleagues stand shoulder to shoulder with you despite the pressure, that's what being *battle-tested* means. It means they've weathered the hard parts of this work, and they don't simply show up, but they help navigate through tricky waters. It's not about being perfect. It's about being proven.

Speaking of battle-tested, it is likely that you, yourself, have not been battle-tested. This leaves you vulnerable, which is exactly why you need a mentor.

The Mentor

In all of this, a mentor is imperative. I wouldn't have made it without mine. He didn't have a stake in the specific fights I was leading. He wasn't trying to take credit. He wasn't trying to climb a ladder.

But time and again, when I was standing on the edge of a decision that could've been a disaster, especially when a trusted colleague turned on me, my mentor was the steady voice that brought clarity. He saw what I couldn't see because he wasn't caught in the emotional fog of the day-to-day. He didn't just teach me tactics, he taught me how to think like a political warrior. He was a guidepost when everything around me felt like it was burning down.

If you can find someone like that, someone outside your organization or team, take the opportunity seriously. They don't have any skin in the game. That space is what gives them clarity.

A true mentor isn't someone who says, "You're doing great!" while you drive off a cliff. A real mentor asks the hard questions. They help you slow down and evaluate without fear or ego. They don't have to be an expert in nursing or the subject matter for the problems you are facing. However, *they must have been through their own fires* and be completely unimpressed by access or proximity to power. They will keep your mission centered and your head clear when lines get blurred.

A good mentor will empathize with the struggle and remind you that deception and poor bargaining are how bad politicians win. They remind you that it means staying true to the mission if you want to see success. If you follow the steps up to this point, you know what you want, have explicitly demanded it, and cannot cave at the first offer thrown at you.

Over the years, I've realized just how rare that kind of mentorship is, and how many nurses never get the guidance they need until it's too late. That's one of the reasons I decided to write this book and create my mentorship program: to give nurses who are ready to lead the kind of practical, real-world support I wish I'd had while at the bedside.

It's not about hand-holding, it's about sharpening. It's about creating change and resuscitating nursing.

The Communicator

The Communicator is among the most underestimated yet vital roles in any advocacy movement. This person is responsible for shaping how your message is received by the outside world and by your own team. A good Communicator doesn't just write well, they *think* well.

When watching for someone to step into this role, look beyond grammar and spelling. Simply being able to use a comma doesn't fit the bill. You will notice the role is "communicator," not writer.

That was intentional.

Look for nurses who know how to read a room. The ones who can adjust their language depending on whether they're talking to staff, patients, or leadership.

Great Communicators often have backgrounds in education, writing, marketing, or even unit-based leadership roles. They're observant, detail-oriented, and they understand the power of tone. They know when to soften and when to strike. Most importantly, they know consistency builds credibility, and sloppy or unclear messaging erodes it quickly.

They can distill complex issues into something that hits hard, reads clearly, and sticks with people. Whether it's a one-pager for a legislator, a social media caption that lights a fire, or talking points for a meeting with administration, the Communicator ensures that what you say reflects what you stand for. They also help prevent confusion and inconsistency across your team's messaging, which is absolutely critical when public pressure begins to build.

If you find someone with a knack for writing and a feel for timing, pull them close. A skilled Communicator will amplify your message, shape your brand, and make sure your movement always sounds like it knows exactly what it's doing.

The Researcher

The Researcher may not be the loudest person in the room, but they're often the reason your message doesn't get shredded in the heat of battle. This role is about more than Googling statistics or printing articles.

The Researcher digs deep for facts, data, policies, and real-world examples. They are the reason your movement isn't just emotional, it's defensible.

When you're looking to fill this role, don't just look for someone who enjoys reading. Look for nurses who ask follow-up questions. The ones who dig into policies "just to be sure." The ones who forward you articles *and highlight what others miss.*

Did you catch that- **they highlight what others miss**. They aren't just throwing information at you. They digest it, connect the dots, and bring you the most crucial information.

Researchers tend to have a touch of healthy skepticism and a drive to understand not just what something *says*, but what it *means*. They notice patterns. They cross-reference sources. Official-sounding statements or buzzwords don't easily fool them.

A strong Researcher knows how to frame evidence in a way that supports strategy. They can pull data that adds weight to your messaging and dismantle opposition spin before it gains traction.

Whether it's reviewing legislation, sourcing historical trends, or building timelines to show systemic failure, the Researcher helps your team put the pieces together and anticipate pushback. They're instrumental in helping your Communicator avoid traps because there's nothing worse than sending out a flashy talking point that falls apart under scrutiny.

If someone on your team has a brain like a filing cabinet and a habit of quietly dismantling propaganda before others catch it, *you've found your Researche*r. Bring them in early, listen when they wave a red flag, and always give them time to verify.

Movements that are grounded in truth win.

Movements that cut corners get buried.

A good researcher keeps you on the right track.

The Sharer

The Sharer takes the message directly to the people. They are your connectors, your educators, your grassroots champions. They may not write the talking points or lead the meetings, but they make sure the message travels.

They tell their friends, talk to their coworkers, and bring the energy to community events. While others may focus on refining the message behind the scenes, the Sharer is busy making sure the message is heard and creating the base to be mobilized.

This role isn't about being loud; it's about being intentional. A strong Sharer knows how to read a room, pick the right words, and deliver the message in a way that makes people *want* to get involved. They're not pushy, but they're persistent. They know how to plant seeds, spark curiosity, and how to open doors without swinging them off the hinges.

Sharers are often nurses who already act as informal educators. You'll notice them calming a patient down with just the right words or turning a 5-minute conversation into a 20-minute mission briefing.

What makes a Sharer truly valuable is their *reach*. They can easily move through personal circles, social networks, and public spaces. They may not see themselves as leaders, but they are the reason movements grow. When people hear others echoing your message, it reinforces credibility.

Why do you think the news channels and papers all repeat the exact words and phrases? The more we hear the message, the more "real" it becomes. Having a handful of quality sharers can ignite untold momentum, and that is power.

If you find someone who genuinely loves talking to people and is passionate about your issue, you've found your Sharer. Equip them with solid messaging, support them along the way, and never underestimate the ripple effect they can create.

The Recon Scout

The Recon Scout quietly monitors political developments, media stories, and internal opposition. They don't speak up often, but when they do, you listen.

Their job isn't to lead or strategize in the open. Their job is to keep your team one step ahead by spotting threats *before* they reach the front line. They're your early warning system for both opportunity and sabotage.

A good Recon Scout has a nose for patterns. They're naturally observant, low-drama, and tend to keep receipts even when no one's asked. You'll recognize them by how they casually mention an issue you hadn't heard of yet, or flag something suspicious in an email that everyone else overlooked. They aren't looking for attention, they're looking for accuracy. And they're rarely wrong.

This role is especially critical when momentum builds and the stakes get higher. Politicians will start whispering, opposition groups will start watching, and internal critics may begin posturing.

Your Scout keeps track of shifting alliances, emerging narratives, and potential vulnerabilities without needing the spotlight. They help you spot infiltration, identify useful intelligence, and understand what the opposition is planning *before* it lands in your lap.

Interestingly, this role may be filled by unexpected helpers. Sometimes, inside leaders, including middle management, will sympathize with the cause and assist you with intel. You must protect their identity if they provide you with quality information and insights. Depending on the information they share with you, they could be risking their jobs.

At the same time, you must not be so eager that you fall for a false friendship. Once you become effective as an advocate for resuscitating nursing, you could find yourself with a "plant" or someone put close to you to "spy." Be especially cautious when new 'scouts' appear at high-stakes moments with insider tips. Things that seem too good to be true often are.

Don't assign this role to someone just because they're good at research or like to gossip. This is a high-trust, low-ego position. Your Scout must be discreet, disciplined, and focused. If you have someone with strong instincts, sharp political radar, and the ability to stay quiet until it matters, pull them in. Just like in the military, good reconnaissance can save a mission before it ever begins.

Flexibility

You don't need a perfect structure to get started. People may move between roles or blend them depending on their skillsets, availability, and the movement's growth. One person might be an excellent researcher and a decent strategist.

Another may begin as a Sharer but grow into an Organizer as their confidence builds. This flexibility is not a weakness. It's actually a strength. It allows you to adapt in real time, to stay lean, and to meet the demands of the moment without building unnecessary hierarchy.

That said, **clarity is still key**. Just because roles are flexible doesn't mean they should be vague. Your team should know what is expected of them. If they're leading communications, they need to be clear that it's their job to create or polish messaging to stay on point so that you can approve and get it out there. If they're organizing meetings, it's their job to follow up on action items and get meeting minutes out if needed. Everyone on your team should have a sense of ownership over their role. Keep the lines of communication open and be honest about when expectations shift or capacity changes. You're not just building a team, you're building a culture of trust, accountability, and shared responsibility. That culture will carry you through battles far more effectively than a polished org chart ever could.

While you will keep a close eye on communications going out, meetings with politicians, and mobilization, you want to ensure that you are working to build up the next generation of leaders. Eventually, you will need to have someone to replace you. This task is much easier when you have a group behind you that is well organized and capable of transitioning roles.

As you build your team, begin scanning your environment for natural allies and inside leaders, as we discussed. Not everyone is ready to join the fight publicly, but that doesn't mean they aren't positioned to help from within. Look for the quiet nurses who know where the bodies are buried, those who've been around, who have institutional knowledge, and know how things work.

Inside leaders may not attend rallies, but they can provide key intel, test ideas, and quietly influence decision-makers behind closed doors.

Likewise, pay attention to those who light up when you talk about change. They're often your natural allies. Don't overwhelm them by dumping a to-do list. Invite them into the process slowly. Ask for feedback. Include them in conversations. Let them build trust through involvement, not pressure. Some will stay on the sidelines, and that's fine. But some will surprise you by stepping up when it matters most.

Networking outside your immediate circle is just as important. Building bridges inside and outside your facility opens up new channels of influence and support.

Professional associations can offer legitimacy and strategic leverage, but be careful. Some are deeply entrenched in systems that resist change. Learn to navigate them with discernment.

More importantly, create secure spaces where you and your team can brainstorm, decompress, and vent. *Privately*. Don't air strategy or frustrations in public forums.

Your credibility is a currency. Spend it wisely. And remember: some of the most valuable collaborations will come from outside nursing altogether.

Hospitals have long used patient advocacy groups to push their agenda. It's time nurses did the same, for the right reasons.

Patients want safe care. We want safe staffing. Those goals are aligned. Strategic collaboration with patient groups not only strengthens your cause but also gives it moral weight that administrators and politicians can't easily dismiss.

While you're at it, get comfortable with the **gray groups**, those who aren't your allies or enemies. Look for groups already fighting for transparency, safety, or autonomy in healthcare.

You don't have to agree on everything. If your values align with the issue at hand, that's enough to work together. Not everyone is going to march with you, and that's okay. Not everyone has to buy into *everything* for you to make progress on *something*. Learn how to work in parallel with others without drama or unnecessary turf wars.

In the end, you are not just organizing people, you are cultivating leadership, strategy, and momentum. Your team doesn't need to be big to be powerful. It needs to be steady, focused, and committed.

You are building a structure that can withstand pressure and grow over time.

Lone warriors may start the fight, but rarely carry it to victory alone. Without a team, your impact is capped, your energy drains faster, and your enemies can isolate you, outlast you, and bury your efforts in red tape and empty promises.

Real change demands a chorus of voices, diverse strengths, and shared resilience. If you want to build something that lasts, you need more than passion.

You need an army.

That army will convert you from a "problem child" to a credible threat when you are able to mobilize your army. But first, you must be able to communicate.

[illegible] soulmate that won't [illegible] hold pass [illegible] grow [illegible]

[illegible]

[illegible] read perspectives.

[illegible]

[illegible]

[illegible]

6
Strategic Communication

*"I think one's feelings waste themselves in words;
they ought all to be distilled into actions
which bring results."
- Florence Nightingale*

Unfortunately, in politics, communication is not just about effectively getting your point across using facts, statistics, and common sense. For the most part, those things matter very little.

You may need to read that again.

For the most part, in battles with politicians, facts, statistics, and common sense do *not* win. They are essential, and you need to have them. But when the rubber meets the road, these things will not cinch victories.

Our skills are based on evidence-based practice and critical thinking, so it can be challenging to understand why these basic principles we rely so heavily on do not work.

The truth is, politics is not about science. It is not about debating over what is right. Usually, it is about money and the opinions of "stakeholders." The nurse and patient rarely fit those categories in a motivating way, which means that we have to find a different way.

If nurses want to win, we must learn how to play the political game. It's a power struggle, who rules whom, and it's pretty dog-eat-dog.

Or do we?

I'll be candid with you. I'm a pretty no-nonsense kind of person. I don't want to play the political game. I don't want to sweet-talk liars, tiptoe around leadership egos, or spend hours in meetings that go nowhere.

I want to sit down, talk about real solutions to complex problems, and do what is ethically correct.

That's why **confrontational politics** works so well for me, and why it works so well for nurses. It isn't politics as usual. It shifts the political game into the world of **negotiation**, and negotiation is something we can master.

The Lost Art of Negotiation

I grew up on a farm. We went to cattle sales. We bought and sold animals. We made deals over tailgates and mucky boots. You learn really fast how to read people. You learn valuation, when to hold firm, and how to walk away if the deal's not right.

That's negotiation.

It's a skill. It's a mindset. And it's something our society doesn't teach anymore.

Unless you were lucky enough to grow up on a farm or in a family business, you may never have experienced high-stakes negotiation in a personal way. That's a disadvantage we carry in modern society. We're trained to accept what we're given. To say thank you and move on.

You don't negotiate the price of bread. You don't haggle at the gas station. You don't argue with your paycheck. It just gets directly deposited. Most of us go through life with very few opportunities to practice negotiation, especially when the stakes are personal.

But here's the problem: hospitals and political systems count on that. They recognize that most people are unaware of how to push back. So when you demand safe staffing, ethical care, or basic human decency, they'll offer you something less, expect a "thank you," and call it a win.

They're playing chess.

So far, you've been playing checkers.

You've been trained to say, "Thank you." It's time to learn to say, "Not enough."

Consumer vs. Political Negotiation: What's the Difference?

Consumer Setting	**Hospital/Political Setting**
Market-driven prices (grocery, gas, utilities)	Negotiable conditions (staffing, policies, budgets)
"Customer is always right" culture	Power hoarding, authority doesn't want to be questioned
Transactions are short-term & impersonal	Decisions affect lives, careers, and patient safety
You can walk away at any time. Shopping elsewhere is easy	You're embedded in the system; you must speak up
Refunds or exchanges are options	Consequences are long-term and systemic

In consumer life, we've been trained to think our only power is to accept or decline.

In hospital life, your power lies in your numbers, your visibility, and your refusal to accept half-steps.

You don't have to be rude.

You don't have to be emotional.

You have to be strategic and speak like a negotiator.

That's why the next part of this chapter will walk you through exactly how to:

- Hold your ground without hostility.
- Frame your expectations without compromise.
- Respond to half-measures with clarity and confidence.
- Keep your message aligned with action and pressure.

This isn't about arguing for the sake of arguing. It's about reclaiming your voice in a system that's conditioned you to stay quiet. Because if they think you'll accept, or approve of, the first low-ball offer, they'll never bring the second one. So, you must hold your ground without hostility.

That leaves us with a big question:

"How do I refuse to compromise while continuing to engage and work towards a goal?"

Unfortunately, there aren't hard and fast rules. This comes with some practice and is more of an art.

When you negotiate with the same people repeatedly, come in with a sound valuation, initiate the negotiation process, and conduct yourself with integrity, your reputation precedes you. You garner respect, and your peers know that you aren't going to try to work them over, and you expect them to hold the same standards.

You might come in with a range of what is acceptable, and you may start your negotiations on the higher end of what you would like, but you walk in knowing your non-negotiables. Your non-negotiables are where you draw the line.

> ***Pro Tip:*** Non-negotiables might include the staff-to-patient ratios, while negotiables might consist of the time frame or manner in which it is done.

Words matter. Think about how management does it. They don't concede; instead, they use gaslighting and continuously shift the blame onto the staff. Now, I am not suggesting that nurses play dirty. I suggest you draw the line in the sand and plant your feet firmly. The best way to do this is by using the REAL Talk Framework. It uses respectful language that neutralizes gaslighting and helps achieve your mission.

REAL stands for:

Step	**What It Means**	**Example Function**
R – Recognize	Acknowledge the effort or gesture	"I appreciate the effort…"
E – Evaluate	Briefly state why it falls short or doesn't meet the need. Provide receipts, too	"…but it doesn't resolve the safety concerns"
A – Assert	Clearly state your non-negotiable expectation	"We need a written commitment to a staffing grid, not a survey"
L – Link Back	Tie the conversation to patient safety, ethics, or SMART-E goals	"Without this, patient outcomes and nurse retention will suffer"

Using the REAL Talk framework, you can quickly plan out phrases before you go into negotiations. However, you can also use it on the fly to ensure you remain professional without losing ground.

Here are a few examples:

1. On Staffing Proposals

"I appreciate your willingness to look into staffing, but evaluating the issue isn't enough. We need a timeline for hiring and a hard ratio. Without that, patient safety is still compromised."

2. On Retention Incentives

"It's good to hear you're offering bonuses, but what we need is workload balance. Bonuses won't keep burned-out nurses here. We need guaranteed shift caps and backup coverage."

3. On New Nurse Orientation Fixes

"I see you've adjusted the orientation length, but unless preceptors are given manageable assignments, it's just lip service. We need protected orientation shifts with clear patient caps."

4. On Intermediate Goals

"Posting open positions is a great first step, but that alone won't improve conditions. Until trained nurses are consistently at the bedside, morale and outcomes will remain at risk."

5. On a Leadership Roundtable Invite

"I appreciate the invite to join the leadership meeting, but real input requires decision-making power. I'm happy to participate if we can agree that nurse feedback will directly influence policy."

6. On a Delayed Response

"Thank you for the update, but progress reports are not a substitute for action. We need a signed implementation plan with dates. Anything less won't earn back our trust."

7. On Deflection or Blame

"I hear this issue has many moving parts, but shifting blame doesn't solve it. Nurses need solutions, not redirection. The accountability lies with leadership, and we expect follow-through."

8. On Token Recognition

"Recognition is appreciated, but what matters most is being heard when we advocate for change. Without staffing reform and support, public praise is hollow."

Let them play their game. You work for *REAL* change.

This framework keeps your message grounded, strategic, and powerful. You're not just reacting emotionally, you're using intentional, prepared language that maintains control of the conversation.

Once you have control, you follow up with consequences for failure to act. If you don't plan to keep politicians accountable, just put this book down and forget about it. Seriously.

If you need a refresher on accountability, revisit "political pain" from chapter two. If you skip this step, your words will be meaningless, and politicians will quickly catch on. Instead of being an agent of change, you will simply be an annoyance. Instead of being viewed as an angry hornet with a painful sting, you will be nothing more than a tiny little fruit fly.

When you successfully utilize the REAL Talk Framework and accountability, politicians will be forced to adopt a different tactic: incrementalism or excuses. We discussed this in Chapter Three and will expand upon it in the next section.

Framing Progress vs. Falling for Incrementalism

You'll shift the power dynamic once you use the REAL Talk Framework paired with accountability. Politicians and hospital leaders will recognize that you're not just venting, you're negotiating.

You're serious.

That's when their tactics shift. If they can't silence you, they'll try to slow you down. Incrementalism becomes their next strategy. They'll offer small gestures. Token changes. Promises to "keep the conversation going." And if you're not prepared, those scraps can start to look like real progress.

This is where your words and how you frame them become your strongest weapon. Remember in Chapter Three we discussed the importance of SMART-E goals? This is why. When your goals are realistic, specific, and measurable, you can easily distinguish between *momentum* and *manipulation.* Sometimes, intermediate goals are necessary, but they should be like mile markers on a road trip, not detours or dead ends.

The key is how you frame the progress: You can acknowledge a step forward without losing sight of the final destination. You can acknowledge a partial win *without declaring victory*. This is where words really matter.

"Posting open positions is a great first step; however, until we have trained nurses at the bedside, patient safety and nurse satisfaction will continue to suffer. We expect…"

That's what this section is about. We will talk about how to frame progress in a way that celebrates steps without settling for less, so you don't get stuck clapping for breadcrumbs while the real reform gets tabled "until next quarter."

Let's make sure your message drives change, not delays it.

Change takes time. Most meaningful victories won't happen overnight. But that doesn't mean we accept *delay* as success or *breadcrumbs as a banquet*. The job of the advocate, especially the front-facing advocate or leader, is to keep the movement focused on the ultimate goal without being dismissive of small steps.

This is where framing becomes your most powerful tool.

It's not just about what you say, it's *how* you say it. You must acknowledge any forward movement without signaling that you are accepting a compromise, or that the offer is "good enough" when it clearly isn't. You must use language that shows strength, not desperation.

Be deliberate about the use of the words acknowledge and accept. Acknowledgment is the recognition of an action. Accepting is the act of agreement with a sense of finality. When intermediate goals are met, you *acknowledge* them. When the goal is met, you *accept* the final result.

Honestly, it is two-fold. You don't want to signal to leadership that you are ready to cave, because as we said, they will make the initial offer and not come back with anything else if they think you will go away. At the same time, your people- your army- they are watching. These words are just as important to them as they are to the politicians you are speaking with.

If you signal that the job is done, or you think the response is good enough, your army will either become demoralized, taking your credibility out the door with them, or worse yet, they may sing the praises of politicians before that credit is due. Sometimes this will cause division in the army, which only leads to more problems.

The more consistent you are, the quicker you will achieve success.

This is still REAL Talk, just adapted for the long game.

- Recognize the step.
- Evaluate its limitations.
- Assert what still must happen.
- Link back to the non-negotiable outcome.

Here are examples of strong framing or holding the line without looking ungrateful:

"That's a step forward. I'll share it with the nurses, but we expect written safe ratios."

"I appreciate the effort, it shows movement. But we're still far from meeting the standards patients deserve."

"That's a gesture, not a solution. Until we see full implementation, we'll keep pressing forward."

"If this is the best you think you can do, I'll inform the staff, but this still falls short of what is needed."

"This will show the nurses that leadership is starting to listen, but still unwilling to take action on what must be done to correct the issue."

"I'm glad to see this step. It signals a willingness to engage, but we still need to see X, Y, and Z."

"Thanks for the update. Please understand, we'll continue organizing until the full standard is met."

These statements maintain a professional tone, clearly communicate expectations, and apply strategic pressure without sounding rude or dismissive.

Pro Tip: If you can tie a law, regulation, or cite a standard from the ANA Nursing Code of Ethics as part of the "L," you will double down on your strength!

Visit https://codeofethics.ana.org/provisions for more information.

Conversely, here are examples of weak framing. They undermine the mission and send the wrong signals. You are telling leadership that the offer is acceptable, you've lowered your expectations, or the issue may no longer be urgent.

Avoid these traps:

> "This is better than nothing."
> *Signals you're grateful for scraps.*
>
> "We're lucky they even responded."
> *Concedes power to leadership and undermines urgency.*
>
> "We can't afford to miss this opportunity."
> *Suggests fear-based acceptance rather than a confident demand.*
>
> "Something is better than nothing, right?"
> *Reinforces the idea that you're negotiable when you're not.*
>
> "At least they're trying."
> *Dilutes pressure and may confuse your team into thinking the goal has changed.*
>
> "We'll take what we can get."
> *Tells leadership they've already won, and they can stop moving.*

If your words aren't clear, consistent, and focused on the goal, you risk sending mixed messages to both the decision-makers and your own team. Framing is your filter. Use it with every response, update, or public statement.

When in doubt, ask:

- *Does this sound like the goal has been achieved, even though it hasn't?*
- *Would a politician walk away from this, thinking they are off the hook?*
- *Would a nurse reading this be tempted to accept what she is given?*

If the answer to any of those is "yes," you must reframe it.

Using this technique is how you stay gracious without giving ground, and it applies to all, no matter who you're speaking to. Different groups respond to different motivators, different language, and different forms of pressure.

If you want to be truly effective, you must add nuance to your communication style, adjusting it without compromising your message. That's what we're going to cover in this next section.

Communicating with Different Audiences

Your advocacy may take you into boardrooms, committee hearings, media interviews, or nurse break rooms. Each setting requires a different approach. This is where we borrow a few tools from our friends in marketing.

If you've never run a side business or worked in branding or advertising, don't worry, but do pay attention. This part matters.

One reliable rule? **Know your audience.**

- **Who am I speaking to, and what role do they play in this issue?**
  (Are they a decision-maker, gatekeeper, ally, or observer?)
- **What motivates them most, power, security, recognition, public image, compliance, or doing the right thing?**
- **What are their pain points, and how does this issue hit them personally or professionally?**
- **Can I connect this issue to their values, emotions, or lived experiences?**
  (People don't move unless they feel something.)
- **Which parts of this message will get their attention, or shut them down?**
  (Look for resistance cues: eye rolls, foot tapping, arms crossed, glazed eyes.)
- **What objections will they raise, and how will I address them without getting defensive?**

- **What words, phrases, or jargon do they use, and how can I mirror them without losing authenticity?**
  (This builds unconscious rapport.)

- **Who or what influences them?**
  (Donors, peers, voters, legal counsel, boards? Speak to those forces when necessary.)

- **How can I frame this so it leads to agreement, or at least action, even if it's just a next step?**

- **What is the one action I want them to take, and how can I make that action feel easy, obvious, and worth it?**

Okay, how do you feel about that?

Do you feel like it is a lot of work? Or do you feel…

Relived?
Focused?
Energized?
Hopeful?

I hope you feel the latter, because using those questions should help remove some of the burden or difficulty of having these conversations. We both know you can never perfectly orchestrate a conversation; you can't predict how others will respond. However, if you answer these questions in advance and understand their perspective, your conversations will become easier. Find these questions and more in your Resuscitating Nursing Workbook and Field Manual.

You have done this before, whether you realize it or not. As nurses, we frequently employ strategic communication, effective questioning, and motivational interviewing techniques. Sometimes, it is working with patients to provide education, behavioral modification, or understanding their history; other times, we use this with physicians when requesting orders. So don't let it intimidate you.

Hospital administrators speak the language of liability, optics, and cost containment. Their pain points usually revolve around lawsuits, staff turnover, budget overruns, and accreditation.

Now let's look at how to apply those questions to real-world conversations with hospital administration, political leaders, the media, fellow nurses, and the public. Each group has different motivators and pain points, meaning your messaging needs to shift without compromising the mission.

They're influenced by legal teams, PR consultants, and corporate executives. When engaging leadership, don't just talk about burnout; talk about *retention* costs. Don't just say "unsafe," say "potential for adverse outcomes that *increase malpractice exposure.*"

Frame your demand as a means to *prevent costly disruption*, and show you've considered implementation. Use their language, *risk mitigation, resource allocation, system strain*, and make your next step easy: "We need a policy change by [X date] to restore trust and ensure compliance."

Legislators care about voter perception, public pressure, and re-election optics. They are influenced by lobbyists, constituents, donors, and party leadership. Motivations vary by party, but no one wants to look incompetent, uncaring, or out of touch. Use stories that connect emotionally *and* represent a broader public trend.

Their pain points? Viral headlines, organized opposition, and reputational damage. Use words like *constituent safety, fiscal responsibility,* and *oversight gaps*. Ask: "Will this help or hurt you in the next election?" Then make the next step easy: "Will you sponsor this amendment?" or "Can we get your commitment in writing today?"

The media wants tension, clarity, and a compelling headline. They don't care about boring policies. They need strong visuals, emotional hooks, and easy-to-quote phrases. You will be quoted, so ensure you are over target and on point. Their pain point is irrelevance; they'll move on quickly if your message isn't timely or engaging.

Speak in sound bites, not monologues. Use vivid language that humanizes the problem: “Nurses are burning out faster than hospitals can hire.” Or: “Patients are crashing while call lights blink unanswered.”

Avoid acronyms or insider language unless you define them. Give them the hook *and* the solution. Next step? “Would you like to speak with a bedside nurse who’s lived this?” or “We’ll email the one-pager with evidence and quotes right after this call.”

Your **fellow nurses** are your base. They already feel the pressure. *Your job is to clarify the solution and show that change is possible.* Their pain points are moral injury, exhaustion, betrayal, and a sense that nothing ever changes.

They’re motivated by protecting patients and restoring their dignity as professionals. Don’t get lost in politics, anchor your message in shared experience: “You know what it’s like when no one comes when ….. That’s what we’re fighting to fix.” Frame the issue as solvable and the demand as doable: “Can we count on you to sign and share this petition?” or “Can you bring one more nurse to the next meeting?”

Your **allies, patient advocates, and the public** may not be in the trenches, but they *care deeply about the impact.* Their pain points are feeling helpless or misinformed. They’re motivated by justice, empathy, and transparency.

Focus on personal stories, ripple effects (e.g., longer ER wait times, delayed discharges), and a clear villain (profit-driven systems, silencing of nurses, etc.). Avoid using jargon; instead, speak in plain terms. “Nurses are being told to care for more patients than is physically possible. It’s not just unsafe, it’s inhumane.” Next step? “Will you speak at the hearing? Share this story? Email your representative?”

Now, with all of that, it is essential to remember these are generalizations. While most of the time they are true, you must remember that people are individuals. The more you can hone in on the individual you are talking to and appeal to their needs, wants, and desires, the quicker your job will be. Falling for generalizations and missing out on individualized conversations are among several pitfalls to which anyone can succumb.

Advocacy Pitfalls

Let's talk a little more about these pitfalls.

Gaslighting is a power play, and hospital leaders and politicians are masters of it. When you are gaslit, immediately pause. Make a note of what buttons you are hitting, because they are working. You should celebrate this victory while listening intently and gathering as much information as possible.

When they switch to gaslighting, they know you have them. Hospital admins will try to convince you that the problem isn't real, that you misunderstood, or that no one else sees it your way. They may even twist your concern into a character flaw:

"You're being dramatic."

"You're the only one complaining."

These tactics are designed to make you question your memory, your motives, or your professional judgment. That's why **receipts matter.**

Documentation, data, emails, meeting notes, staffing logs, direct quotes, timelines, these are your protection. But even more than that, they're your power. A well-documented concern becomes harder to deny. A pattern backed by evidence is more complicated to dismiss. Having a plan and the paper trail to support it allows you to push past gaslighting attempts and redirect the conversation back to the issue and your proposed solution.

Your job isn't to convince them you're "nice" or "reasonable." Your job is to stay rooted in reality and push for meaningful action. This is where a mentor can come in handy. You may be tempted to hop on the explanation train or cower in embarrassment.

DON'T DO IT.

You have the moral high ground. STAND FIRM and make sure you push those same buttons that resulted in the gaslighting. Your techniques are working.

> ***Pro Tip:*** This is often called "doubling down," meaning that you double your efforts, you repeat the phrases that caused the reaction, only bigger, stronger, and faster.

In the aftermath of gaslighting, or at other points during your mission, you may be tempted to over-negotiate. Especially when politicians pretend to compromise or throw out phrases like, *"We just need to meet halfway."*

This is a trap.

If you walk in demanding a 4:1 patient ratio and let them drag you to 6:1 "just to get something done," you've compromised your entire mission.

You will have taught them that your demands are soft.

That you will crumble under a little pressure, and they will use this to demoralize your army.

That's where SMART-E goals protect you. They aren't just about being realistic, they're about being **anchored**. If your goal is specific, measurable, and built around a meaningful effect, there's no reason to entertain vague alternatives or watered-down language.

Negotiation should never be a slow slide into acceptance. It should be a straightforward, strategic process rooted in what will actually fix the problem. Don't start with your ideal and *hope* to land at a compromise. Start with your non-negotiable, and defend it as the common-sense solution that it is.

But holding your ground isn't just about what you say in the room. It's about what you do afterward. Advocacy requires more than powerful words. No one wants a leader who likes to hear themselves talk and fails when it's time to deliver. It doesn't matter how passionate your speech is, how viral your post goes, or how many people nod along in the meeting. **If your words aren't backed by consistent action, your credibility dissolves, and your movement stalls.**

This doesn't mean you have to do everything yourself. But it does mean your message needs to match your behavior. If you say unsafe staffing is an emergency, don't turn around and celebrate the formation of yet another vague "staffing task force." If you demand patient-centered care, don't endorse leadership initiatives that exclude nurses from the conversation.

People are watching what you say, and what you do after you say it. Say less and do more, or make sure what you say is what you *plan to make real*. Otherwise, you're not advocating. You're performing.

This can also be tricky when you have built a team, not so much that your words and actions are inconsistent, but that the messaging can shift when multiple people are advocating. Even a slight deviation can cause you, or your team, to lose focus, momentum, and credibility.

This is called **message drift**, which happens when different advocates start "freelancing" their wording, tone, or goals. One person softens the demand to sound more agreeable. Another exaggerates the threat. Another contradicts the goal because they didn't fully understand it. Suddenly, leadership is confused, your base is scattered, and your opponents exploit the inconsistency.

The solution? Assign a communicator and make sure written communications pass through you. As discussed in Chapter Five, this person ensures that everything going out, press statements, social posts, and meeting talking points, is clear, unified, and aligned with your SMART-E goals. A consistent message is more complicated to twist, easier to repeat, and more likely to earn support.

Drift weakens movements.

Clarity wins.

Closing Thoughts on Strategic Communication

Strategic communication is not about sounding good; it's about being effective. In the world of politics and hospital power structures, emotional appeals and moral authority are not enough. You need a plan, a message, and the discipline to deliver both consistently. The tools in this chapter exist to protect your mission and amplify your voice without compromise.

You now know how to frame progress without sacrificing your goals. You've learned to speak to different audiences in their language, without losing your own. And you've been warned of the pitfalls: gaslighting, over-negotiating, hollow messaging, and message drift. These are traps designed to slow you down or fracture your movement. But they only work if you let them.

"Your words are your scalpel. Use them to cut through excuses and expose the heart of the problem."

Keep your communication focused. Stay grounded in your goals. Speak like someone who knows what's at stake, because you do.

You don't need to be polished. You don't need to be perfect.

But you do need to be clear, consistent, and unshakably committed.

If you can do that, no politician, hospital executive, or PR team will be able to silence you. The people watching, the nurses behind you, and the patients depending on you will know exactly who to follow.

You don't just speak for yourself anymore. You speak for the change that's coming.

Let's Resuscitate Nursing.

Closing Thoughts on Strategic Communication

[illegible]

7
Mobilization
What It Is and What It Isn't

"Unnecessary noise is
the most cruel absence of care
that can be inflicted on the sick."
- Florence Nightingale

It's time to move!

You've made it this far. You've named the problem, picked your battle, laid out your SMART-E goals, clarified your messaging, and started building your team. Now comes the pivot. It's time to move.

It's time to mobilize.

But let's pause for a moment. What does that even mean? We throw the word around a lot. "Mobilize the base." "Mobilize your network." "Mobilize for change."

But if you don't know what mobilization actually is, you're going to waste a whole lot of energy, and you'll walk away burned out, confused, and wondering why no one showed up.

Mobilization isn't just movement. It's a *directed* movement. It's the difference between a flash mob and a firing squad. One looks exciting. The other gets results.

Before you can mobilize effectively, you must understand what specific change you're after. There are two kinds: **grassroots** and **institutional**.

Grassroots change begins with everyday people, including nurses, patients, and families, pushing from the outside. It's public, it's loud, and it applies pressure.

Institutional change comes from within: committee discussions, policy revisions, and administrative shifts. It sounds more professional, but here's the catch: **institutional change only moves when the system wants to move.**

Grassroots change? It moves when the people say *enough*.

Spoiler alert: that's the one that works.

Institutional change is slow, polite, and easily absorbed. When done right, grassroots change **creates public pressure that cannot be ignored.** It doesn't ask for permission. It makes the price of ignoring you too high. It forces decision-makers to act not because they want to, but because they no longer have a choice.

That's what this chapter is about. Not waiting. Not asking nicely. **Mobilizing**.

This is the distinction that separates effective advocates from those who are exhausted.

Institutional change is safe. It plays by the rules of the system. You'll sit on a task force, submit a proposal, or give input in a roundtable, only to find that nothing really changes. The system absorbs it. The urgency gets buried in bureaucracy. And leadership pats themselves on the back for listening.

Grassroots change doesn't wait to be invited. It simply shows up. It calls out excuses. It doesn't accept delays as progress. It leverages the voice of the people to overwhelm the comfort of power. And yes, it's uncomfortable, even confrontational at times. That's the point.

We're not here to be disruptive or just to make noise. We're disruptive **because disruption is the only thing that moves power when it's stuck.**

Institutional change can matter, but only if the grassroots momentum is strong enough to keep it accountable. If you want policy changes, force a conversation. If you want leadership to act, make the alternative worse than saying no.

So ask yourself: are you here to participate, or are you here to pressure?

If you're ready to pressure, keep reading.

> ***Pro Tip:*** Sometimes politicians will want you to think that institutional change works by moving your ideas through "appropriate channels," i.e., committees. However, we know the truth: the institutional wheels wouldn't have started moving without grassroots pressure.

What Mobilization Isn't

Let's start by clearing the air: most people get mobilization wrong.

Mobilization is not just making noise. It's not showing up angry at a meeting. It's not creating a Facebook group and venting in the comments. It's not going viral with a trending hashtag, and thinking that counts as pressure.

Mobilization isn't awareness.

Awareness is marketing. Mobilization is action.

Social media can be a great tool. It can spread your message, recruit supporters, and expose problems. But if your strategy ends at "raising awareness," you're not doing advocacy. You're doing PR.

The same goes for email campaigns. If you're just writing emails to express frustration or ask for vague "support," don't expect results. Politicians get thousands of emails. They ignore the ones that are polite and forgettable. They act on the ones that are organized, specific, and come with consequences.

Proper mobilization is layered. It begins with a clear demand-your SMART-E goal. Then it stacks pressure via calls, letters, petitions, testimony, visibility, and confrontation. It escalates when necessary. It builds when ignored. It doesn't let go until the demand is met.

If you want your movement to be effective, you must stop thinking like a content creator and start thinking like a tactician. You're not here to make noise. You're here to make them *move*.

Let them wonder what's coming next. Let them feel the discomfort of inaction.

Credibility: Setting the Groundwork

Before you can mobilize others, you must be someone worth following.

Let that sink in.

Mobilization starts with **credibility**, not charisma. You don't need a polished background or fancy title. What you need is actions that are consistent with your words. If nurses don't believe you're in it for the right reasons, if they sense ego or empty ambition, you're done. You can't lead a movement if no one trusts you to finish what you start.

Nurses are sharp. We assess for a living. We watch for inconsistencies, we recognize when people are faking it, and we know when someone's just trying to build a name off other people's pain. If your advocacy is only visible when it benefits you, people will notice, and they'll walk.

Your credibility isn't built in conference rooms with administrators. It's built in the trenches. It's the long nights digging through policies, the early mornings writing handouts no one sees, the consistent follow-up after the spotlight fades. It's refusing to roll over when it gets hard. It's picking up the phone when you'd rather be anywhere else.

That's where leadership is proven.

In the first course I took, they likened an effective grassroots leader to a general charging the hill, leading the charge from **the front lines.** That's what builds trust. That's how you prove you're not just another self-appointed voice.

Initially, you will bear the weight. If you can't handle it, if you dodge responsibility, or only show up for the stage, you won't be followed.

If you say you're going to do something, *do it.*

If you make a mistake, *own it.*

You don't have to be perfect. If you act like you are, nurses will stop listening. But if you're honest when you screw up, if you stay steady when it's messy, if you keep showing up even when you're tired and outnumbered, that's when people start leaning in. That's when the movement gets legs.

Credibility isn't a credential. It's a reputation earned through consistency, integrity, and grit. The more you stay grounded, the more people will trust your leadership, even if they're not ready to speak out themselves, and your movement will grow like wildfire.

Credibility is the first campaign, and the one you never stop running.

Direction is Essential

The number one reason most advocacy efforts fail?

The people don't know what they're asking for.

Don't expect anyone to act if your "call to action" is vague, emotional, or scattered. People don't follow confusion. They follow clarity.

You cannot mobilize around a feeling. You must mobilize around a **demand**.

You will pull from Step One, Identifying the Problem, and your SMART-E goal. Your demand must be specific, measurable, and action-driven. It must be written down. It must be short enough to say in one breath. And it must be repeated so often that your team says it in their sleep.

This is where many nurses go wrong. They start making noise without naming a target. They go on social media rants or attend board meetings and unload a list of grievances. And yes, it's tempting. It feels cathartic. But you're not here to vent. You're here to win. And no one wins a war when the troops don't know what hill they're charging.

"Simply whacking the hornets' nest and creating a swarm is not enough to create change. You must ensure the swarm knows the target and can go after it."

Mobilization without direction is chaos.

Mobilization with a clear demand is power.

That demand becomes your rallying cry. It becomes the heartbeat of your movement. Whether it's "pass this bill," "drop this mandate," "publish this data," or "implement a minimum staffing ratio," it needs to be laser-focused and impossible to misinterpret.

During your campaign, and through the various phases, you must effectively communicate your expectations to your army and WHY they must be carried out.

One of my biggest pet peeves is a leader who expects people to follow them, no questions asked. Don't just tell people what to do. **Tell them why it matters**.

Nurses are critical thinkers. We don't follow blindly. And frankly, **we shouldn't**. One of the biggest red flags in leadership is someone who expects blind loyalty without transparency. Your job is not to bark orders, it's to make the mission clear, relevant, and urgent.

That's how you earn trust and **keep your army aligned and engaged.**

Part of the reason nursing is such a mess is that we have been battered and bruised into submission. We, as nurses, have carried burdens imposed by poor management practices and unrealistic expectations. We have just accepted poor conditions and policies devoid of morals. Now, at a time when change seems futile, busy nurses are not going to invest a lot of time. They are not going to read a dissertation on your cause. They're not going to decode a 600-word paragraph buried in passive language. If your message isn't crystal clear by the second sentence, you've already lost most of your audience.

So what do you do?

You keep it simple for most people in the army, but you make additional information about the problem and your SMART-E goal available; however, don't overwhelm people with information.

In a call to action, you keep it tight. You keep it simple. And you communicate one step at a time.

Not the following five steps.

Not your grand vision for six months from now.

Just the next step.

What needs to be done *right now?*

So here is the format I use to mobilize. You've likely seen versions of this if you've followed any serious grassroots campaign. Why? Because it works. It's fast, direct, and respects people's time and energy. I call it the WISAL. Because like a whistle chirps, clear and usually causes people to move.

W - Who you are
I - Issue at hand
S - Solution for the issue
A - Action that must be taken & when
L - Learn more

WISAL Messaging

1. Who you are: "This is [Name] with [organization name]
2. The issue is: ____________________
3. The Solution is: ____________________
4. You need to [take this ACTION] by [date/time] and say "____________"
5. Learn- Get more info [provide a link or method to obtain more info] and encourage them to share feedback with you.

First of all, each of these steps will be a singular sentence, maybe two sentences for number four, but seriously, keep this super short.

In your text, you always want people to know it is you- if they know and trust you, they will keep reading. Also, this is required if you are using a texting service, so you may as well get used to adding it.

Next, you will state the issue in a brief, direct way. The issue or problem should be clear, so the solution is actionable and obvious based on your SMART-E goal. Then you need to give the explicit instructions, ensuring there is a deadline for action and a short, strong, repeatable phrase they can use.

You might feel a little bossy or bold doing this, but honestly, it was one of the best choices I made in my advocacy. The number one complaint I heard from people is "I just don't know what to say."

Think about it. They are rarely subject matter experts and might even get nervous about taking action. Again, this isn't business as usual. This is a demanding change to a system that is designed to control. Most people will appreciate the guidance; those who don't want to use it won't. For the most part, that is ok.

Finally, the last line, sharing additional info as well as requesting feedback...

Inevitably, some people will have more questions, so it can be helpful to direct them back to a website or social page where they can get more details. Honestly, there was a point in my advocacy work where this was burning me out.

You'll have people who want details. They'll want to understand every angle before taking action. That's fine, but your time is better spent leading than repeating yourself twenty times.

This is where a centralized info hub saves you.

Whether it's a simple website, a password-protected page, a pinned post on social, or a shareable Google Doc, create a place where your army can get answers without needing to come back to you directly.

You're not giving away your strategy there. You're giving your team what they need to feel confident taking action:

- The backstory (brief)
- The goal (clear)
- Talking points or FAQs
- Contact info or links

When you drop a WISAL with a link to this resource, you don't have to stop and answer the same 15 questions. You just say, "Full info is at the link." That alone will save you hours and keep the focus where it belongs, on the mission.

Encouraging feedback doesn't mean opening the floodgates for personal critiques on your style or leadership. Typically, your call to action will result in people interacting with decision-makers (i.e., politicians). Even if they are communicating with the decision-maker's secretary, you can garner a lot of information about how well the pressure is working or even a new pain point.

This information is a powerful resource you want to tap into, and you can also use it as encouragement in your next call to action. Inviting feedback creates a sense of connection between you and your army, and that what they do is essential. This reinforces trust, transparency, and morale.

> ***Pro Tip:*** Your job is not to control everything, and it will be vital that you don't get caught up in everyone being precisely the same. Believe me, sometimes these alterations make all the difference and lead to gaining vital information. There's a difference between independent thinkers and those actively undermining your mission. The first group makes you stronger. The second makes you unstable. If someone's off-script but still pushing toward the same goal, keep them close. But if they're eroding trust or sowing confusion, it's time to let them go. Talk to your mentor. Trust your gut. Protect the movement.

> ***Pro Tip:*** When you consistently keep your info accessible, people start using it automatically. You've trained your army to look for answers *before* coming to you. That's how you scale. That's how you stay sane.

Layers of Mobilization: How Pressure Builds

Once you've earned credibility and established a clear demand, it's time to **turn up the heat**. This is where mobilization becomes tactical.

You don't just throw everything at the wall and hope something sticks. You build pressure in layers, each one louder, sharper, and more public than the last. And each one is designed to make one thing clear:

"We are not going away and will hold you accountable."

Accountability will be key at every step of this process. Much like nursing, if it wasn't documented, activism wasn't done.

That means all interactions with politicians are documented. Any receipts that you can collect will be to your benefit. Sometimes, receipts come in the form of emails, bulletins, quotes from public meetings, and even sometimes, phone calls.

But here is the thing: if a promise wasn't public or in writing, it doesn't count. It becomes your word against theirs. So, when it is crucial, ensure there are witnesses or some form of documentation. Sometimes, I will follow up with personal conversations through email and request a response. That way, I can show commitment or the failure to do so.

Just remember, keep documentation of everything, and ensure it is kept on your personal devices or paper that you can take with you and store in a secure location. Losing the war because you can't access your receipts would be a terrible tragedy.

Below, I am going to outline a general theme of tactical escalation. However, there are times when you will bounce between these depending on the situation and flow of the mission. For some of these tactics, you will need to discern whether you should be leading from the front, like the general charging the hill, or if you should be "leading from the rear." That means there will be times in the war when you cannot afford to be on the front lines and vice versa.

When you are playing chess with politicians, you can't afford to be taken off the board. Discern when you not only can, but *should* drop back in the ranks and allow the mass and weight of the army to do the heavy lifting.

Ultimately, it is your ability to mobilize effectively that will win the war, not your voice alone. Ego and pride can trick us into thinking that we must always stand at the front; however, if you become a martyr for the cause, who will lead? So be sure to discern these situations.

Petitions & Signature Collection

Petitions and signature collections are your basic layer of army building. Petitions provide a list, and that list gives you leverage. But don't just collect signatures for the sake of optics.

Collect **contact info and follow up**.

This is how you build your base and grow your army for future action. No petition should ever end with a "thank you." It should always end with: "What can you do next?" You should think of the petition as an invitation. When they list their email or phone number, they are essentially saying, "Yes, I want you to keep me informed."

Surveys may play a similar and essential role in building your army, but also in finding out what is important to them and aiding in picking the proper fight at the right time.

Personal Letters & Testimony

These hit hard, but rarely make an impact. You probably think you know where I am going…

"Ok, a single heartfelt story may be overlooked. We just need more, a dozen stories, printed and hand-delivered with specific requests? That turns heads, right? We will ensure they're personalized, short, and clearly repeat the demand. Then we coordinate delivery, and the politician will beg for a meeting."

Wrong.

That's where most people go *wrong*. While personal stories are filled with heartbreak and the desperate hope for change, they rarely sway politicians. They may feel a momentary twinge of morals, but when it comes down to it, they won't change their direction.

So, you are probably wondering why I included this.

First, you will document the responses they give you and have others do the same. Collect this information and keep it safe with your receipts.

This is an obligatory step. Do not anticipate any change. Act with integrity and allow politicians to do the right thing.

Do not have high expectations. Be ready to read between the lines, and get sympathetic puppy dog eyes at most. Remember that sympathy is not the same thing as action.

When you don't see any action, remember…

These stories aren't for the politician- they are for the people. The politicians might be the ones they are addressed to, but personal stories are really intended for your fellow nurses, the patients, the public, and the media.

Confusing- I get it. Feels a bit underhanded? No, because you hope that they will take action. The politician has the opportunity to act, change course, and do the right thing. However, you must be prepared for the reality that it won't work.

In these instances, you must use pressure to elicit a response. Once the letters are delivered, the job is not to sit back and wait.

These stories are being shared to provoke change, and it is your responsibility to use them for such.

Obviously, you will get permission from the writer to share their stories. This may include interviews, publishing the letters, or social media graphics. The goal here is to expose how these problems harm people and how your mission is to correct these wrongs.

Sharing these emotional stories, exposing the fact that the politicians are aware, and yet continue to be unwilling to take action, grabs the media's attention, and it is a PR nightmare for the hospital.

The bottom line is that, if you are asking people to take the time to write a letter, maximize their efforts. Don't just let it be delivered to the politician who will promptly file it in the "circular file" (paper shredder). Let their voice be heard through your own releases or the media.

> ***Pro Tip:*** Be cognizant of legal traps and violations of confidentiality. Sharing stories from nurses is one thing; however, if you are sharing the experience of a patient, then you may want to consult with legal counsel. At the very minimum, get a release signed. There will be an example of a generic release in your Resuscitating Nursing Workbook and Field Manual or in the resources at wtajourney.com/rnworkbook, but be advised- I am not an attorney. I am not your attorney. I am not giving legal advice. The resource is a starting point. You are responsible for reviewing that release with your legal counsel.

Calls & Emails: Timed and Targeted

Emails are some of the easiest mobilization tools that can be used. They are quick and direct. I will be honest, though. In my opinion, calls are much more effective.

Emails are easy, relatively quick, and can be made in template format. Depending on your resources, the size of your organization, or the level at which you are engaging, there may even be software that your army can plug in their information and automatically send a form email.

Of course, this removes the excuse of being busy. It is effortless for the individual to do because they don't have to think. They punch in their information and hit send.

Sounds great…

I see a couple of drawbacks. First, these people are barely engaged. They aren't likely to build up into the next layer if this is the most they can do. It gives them an excuse not to take any additional steps.

Secondly, these form emails with standard subject lines *might* get counted before the staff member hits DELETE. Even if the individual took the time to write something personal in the body, the staff member isn't likely to get that far. Any additional time spent is likely wasted.

From my experience with legislators, I have found that they often use automated responses that can demoralize activists. The activists may feel that you asked them to do something with the intent to make a change, only to receive a generic email or letter in return. The blame may not lie with the politician, but rather on your shoulders because you asked the activist to take meaningless action.

Yikes! So, if you use mass email messages, be prepared for this possibility. Encourage the activists to reach out via phone or a second email requesting a personal response. These types of interactions can also be added to your receipts file!

Third, most companies that do these automated emails are data-mining.

What will they do with the data that your army shares with them?

Will they collect donations?

Will they use it to target them in some way? Perhaps through advertisements or propaganda?

Will they sell that information to employers, political parties, or others?

I am not saying this is never an option, but just be aware of unintended consequences. The benefits might outweigh the risks for large movements, such as national-level movements.

For small groups, you might draft an email and make it available for people to use, but again, the likelihood that these will have an impact is LOW.

You will have to gauge each situation to determine if this kind of action is warranted. Consider the risks, benefits, and alternatives, then decide what to do. I am not saying that there is never a time and place. I don't want you to be fooled by *passive activism* and "the way everyone else does it." **Emails are a building point, not something that wins the race.** It is a layer of pressure. If you keep that in mind, you will not fall into the trap of passive activism and be left wondering why your tactics are not working.

One of my favorite legislative tactics is the phone call. For me, it works very well.

Our legislators have aids that assist them with drafting bills, scheduling meetings, talking with lobbyists, and more. These aids are sometimes much more knowledgeable about the bills and legislative processes than legislators are. What that means is that these legislative aids are imperative to the workflow of the legislature, and if they are tied up with phone calls, they can't get their other work done. The workflow of legislators is significantly impacted.

They are the direct line to the legislator and also to leadership. That means when they are being pressured and told the same thing over and over again, they will pass it along to the legislator and leadership, which can lead to internal struggle between the individual legislators and leadership.

It also may provide legislators with the "steady ground" to stand on. Meaning that *if* they are inclined to follow the requests of the people, they can point back to the phone calls and all the attention to the issue. Legislative aids may also get frustrated on phone calls and argue or give other information, which can be helpful as you plan and move forward.

Again, disgruntled interactions and any information offered are all receipts and talking points. Sometimes I use them during a phone call campaign, and at other times I hold tight to the information and use it at an opportune time.

While you may not be dealing with legislators, don't underestimate the opportunity that arises with something as seemingly powerless as a secretary. In activism within the hospital, this may or may not be an option for you due to the risk to your job. These things may need to come from outside the hospital, like an advocacy group.

A text service is one of the most effective ways to disseminate information about making phone calls. This allows for a coordinated effort and a high reach rate for your army. I always use the mobilization format, regardless of whether I am pushing a call or email campaign.

We can discuss this further in the infrastructure chapter.

In-Person Presence

This is where you turn discomfort into pressure. Show up at the committee hearing. Attend the hospital board meeting. Be visible, be composed, and be consistent.

The key here is repetition. One appearance can be ignored. A consistent presence fosters a fear of public accountability. Consistent presence also tells you how things are moving forward, what areas you need to monitor for concerns, and more. There is a lot to be gained by simply being present.

However, you can also turn presence into a power play…

Have you ever been to a staff meeting where one dissenting voice, followed by a second, turned a relatively calm group into a pack of rabid wolves? Those organizing the meeting, maybe even you, didn't see it coming, and it happened so fast that there was very little that could be done to stop it.

You can use this momentum to quickly turn a meeting meant for appeasement or control into a defining moment for your cause.

Believe me, it doesn't have to be ugly. With the right tone and pointed questions, you can gain scores of new army members or have the politicians on their heels, making public promises to a room full of people.

Let's go back and think about that staff meeting I spoke of at the beginning of the book. I was one dissenting voice. I could stand my ground firmly and certainly got the CEO on his heels. However, he was able to recover and divert quickly.

If I had a few friends sitting beside me nodding, they wouldn't have made much of a difference. Some people paying attention might have also nodded along, but it likely wouldn't have inspired courage or further dissent.

However, one of the tactics I learned in that initial political course was using the "diamond formation" and how it is used to take over meetings. If I had known and applied this technique, I am sure the CEO would have felt significantly more pressure to change, and we would have inspired others to act as well.

The Diamond Formation is a simple, calculated strategy rooted in psychology, designed to create the illusion of widespread agreement and build pressure through layered, directional influence.

Like I said, you don't want to show up with a couple of friends and sit together. That's not a threat. That's a clique. A group clustered together can easily be dismissed as troublemakers. But people start paying attention when you're spread throughout the room, when it sounds like dissent is coming from all directions. And more importantly, they start joining in.

Here's how it works.

Before the meeting or rally, you and three to seven allies gather to review the likely talking points and rehearse your own. You don't need a script, you need **clarity**. Identify your core message. Then assign roles. Again, your Resuscitating Nursing Workbook and Field Manual are several helpful resources, with a few in the free resources on wtajourney.com/rnbook.

You'll start with what we call **The Initiator**. This is the person who opens the exchange. They're confident, calm, and direct. They raise the first objection or ask the first tricky question, something based on fact, designed to make the speaker slightly uncomfortable, but not combative. Their goal is to shift the tone of the meeting. A good initiator is the match that lights the fuse. Their job is to create the opening, *not* to carry the whole conversation.

Once the Initiator speaks, the others come in, not as a group, but from scattered points in the room. That's where the formation gets its name. While it doesn't need to be perfect, the idea is to form a loose diamond with each participant positioned in a different area of the audience. Think front, sides, and back, not the corners or wallflowers, but intentionally interwoven within the crowd.

Next comes **The Reinforcer**. This person gives nonverbal signals of agreement, such as nodding, leaning in, and making quiet affirmations like "Exactly" or "That's right." They may softly repeat a key phrase from the Initiator's question or say something aloud, just loud enough for surrounding attendees to hear. They're validating the first speaker, building credibility, and priming others to start nodding along.

After that, **the Echo** speaks up. They don't start a new topic; they extend the original concern. Most likely, they will ask for clarification on an evasive answer or offer another example from their own experience supporting the Initiator's point. This is what makes the dissent contagious. Suddenly, it's not just one nurse with a complaint. It's two, three, four, all articulating variations of the same concern. The audience begins to shift.

And then, when the tension is rising, **The Closer** steps in. This is the person who delivers the sharpest point. *They don't raise their voice, but they do ask the most serious question, the one that corners the speaker and demands a public commitment.*

They might reference a specific report or public record or say, "Can we count on [the desired action] within [a time frame]?" The goal is not to get a yes. It's to **force a visible response**, and let the room decide if it's acceptable.

Throughout this process, **Floaters** play a subtle but critical role. They don't speak publicly. Instead, they're scattered among the attendees, making side comments, affirming what's said, and engaging quietly with those around them. They may whisper, "She's right, you should've seen what happened last shift," or respond with concern when someone brushes it off. Their job is to move the room emotionally, to normalize dissent, and to pull others into agreement before they even realize they've joined a movement.

This technique doesn't require theatrics. It requires planning, coordination, and tone. Truthfully, it can happen without a plan, just well-informed team members and a bit of luck.

How do I know?

I have done it. It is probably one of my favorite moments in activism.

I was green in politics and trying to figure things out along the way.

A friend and I attended a meeting hosted by an ally group. They set it up for the legislators, who were dropping the ball and being called out for it. They intended to garner public praise and smooth things over for the politicians. I had only one other person on my team, and they weren't exactly prepared to take action, but they were there to pass around a clipboard and collect signatures.

I was the instigator and started with a strong question. My teammate acted as a floater, charging the room with emotion. A legislator fired back at me, and I made eye contact with a stranger across the room.

HE KNEW THE ASSIGNMENT.

Suddenly, he was sewing dissent, and at that point, the train not only left the station but was barreling off the tracks as two or three other people piped up. There was no way the legislators could recover.

I got lucky that day. The pieces just fell into place, trust me, it doesn't always happen like that.

Diamond formation done well will result in the speaker losing control of the meeting before they realize it. That is exactly what happened that day. The audience will become the voice of accountability, and your team will have lit the spark.

But don't stop there.

Never let an opportunity go to waste.

One of the most common mistakes I see is showing up strong and then leaving empty-handed. You must **convert the moment into momentum**.

In that instance with the hospital CEO, I had no clue about collecting names, building a movement, or that this was even possible. Had I known these things, my outcome might have been vastly different.

However, at the meeting with the legislators, I knew why I was there. I came prepared, and you should too!

As the meeting adjourns and people begin to shuffle out, this is your final opportunity. Assign one or two trusted teammates to wait by the exits. The goal here is to get the contact information of as many people as possible.

I would recommend using a mix of tactics. Some people will take your clipboard and give you their info. Others will be skeptical, so you need a way to connect with them.

You can hand out a quarter-page summary of your goal or demand.

Offer a QR code that leads to an online list builder.

Most importantly, ask the question:

"Do you want to help make this happen?"

Obviously, you can use a variation of the question, but make sure it garners buy-in and promotes action.

You've already done the hard part. You turned the room. Now you capture the energy and **grow your army**.

This isn't just presence. It's precision. It's planning. And it's how you turn a boring agenda into a battleground, and a crowd of silent observers into a coalition for change.

Public Accountability: Receipts Are Your Weapon

There will come a point in every campaign when polite pressure stalls. The meetings are over. The talking points have been exchanged. The smiling nods and vague assurances have worn thin. Now it's time to escalate.

You don't escalate with more noise.

You escalate with receipts.

At this point in your campaign, you've likely gathered stories, submitted letters, organized petitions, attended meetings, and logged dozens of hours on calls and emails.

And, if you followed the advice in previous chapters, you kept a paper trail. You've tracked promises. You've documented responses or silence. This is not about speculation or emotion. You've built a file. Now it's time to put it to use.

This is the moment where public accountability becomes your sharpest tool.

Start publishing what you've documented. Pull quotes from emails, letters, and meeting minutes, and screenshot comments.

Pair promises with the failure to act. Use side-by-side comparisons, timelines, and even short video clips when applicable. You don't have to sensationalize; you have to expose their actions, or inaction.

"On March 2, Hospital Administration committed to upholding staffing grids.

On May 15, they told us it was 'no longer a priority.'

Meanwhile, nurses are still carrying 8:1 med-surg loads. Still losing patients. Still drowning.

Receipts below. You decide."

This isn't a tantrum. It's a tactic.

You're not here to humiliate; you are simply being objective. You're here to remove the excuse of ignorance and create pressure that makes inaction more uncomfortable than taking corrective action. That's what gets results.

Make their silence loud.

If they didn't respond to your petition?
Post that.

If they ignored a mother's letter about a preventable injury?
Post that, with her permission.

If a politician gave a smile and handshake in the room, then voted against you two days later?
Post that, and tag them.

Call the media, but don't show up empty-handed. Bring your timeline, bring your quotes, bring your case. You are not asking for attention. You are providing the truth.

You are doing the job others refuse to do.

In doing all this, you must be sure you are not just pointing out the failures. **You always close the loop.**

Make sure you are pointing back to the action or demand. You must be sure that there is no question about what you expect to happen.

Remember the work from Chapter Three, your SMART-E goal.
Remember the Strategic Triage Framework in Chapter 4.
Remember why you chose this fight.

Now you close the loop.

"We demanded ____.
We offered testimony.
We gathered support.
We followed the process.
They still refused."

This is where your documentation becomes your weapon. You're not just holding politicians accountable, you're showing the public how hard you tried before going public. That matters. You tried to play nice. They played games. Now the audience sees the game for what it is.

You don't have to wait for someone to give you a platform. You've been building one this whole time. Whether it's social media, a letter to the editor, a press release, or a live-streamed community event, use the tools you have at your disposal.

Before moving on to the next section, remember: Mobilization isn't a checklist. It's a dynamic strategy. Each layer, whether it's petitions, personal testimony, phone calls, in-person presence, or public accountability, plays a distinct role in building pressure and shifting power. Sometimes they stand alone; other times, they compound for maximum effect.

What matters most is that you engage with intention. You gather receipts. You stay ready to escalate. And you never let a tactic go to waste. Mobilization isn't about volume. It's about precision, credibility, and persistence. When done right, it becomes undeniable. You're not just speaking up. You're leading a movement that refuses to be ignored.

Overcoming Resistance

If you're doing this right, resistance shouldn't come as a surprise. It's confirmation.

Do you remember in Chapter Two, when we discussed political response and how, if you are being ignored, you are doing it the wrong way?

I will not belabor the point, but I want to remind you that you will face difficulty.

Expect stall tactics. Expect gaslighting. Expect bad-faith actors pretending to be "on your side" while actively undermining your efforts. These aren't signs of failure. They're signals that you're applying real pressure. If you have made it this far in the book, you know it will happen.

What should you do when it shows up?

- **Get louder, not softer**. If they ask you to "tone it down," it means the message is hitting.
- **Repeat the demand**. Don't get dragged into side issues. Don't let them reframe it. Say it again, louder and clearer.

- **Stay public**. They'll try to take the conversation offline, behind closed doors. Be polite, but bring it back to the open where it's accountable.
- **Watch your flanks**. Internal critics will show up when momentum builds. Some will say you're being too harsh. Others will ask for unity. If it distracts from the mission, **stay on target**.
- If needed, review Chapters 2 and 6 for specific pointers.

One of the best pieces of advice from HL Richardson's Confrontational Politics is this: *"The opposition will always try to change the subject. Don't let them."*

Every time they resist, double down on your demand. Pressure causes discomfort; that's the point. You're not here to be managed. You're here to be effective.

Final Rallying Charge

Mobilization is not about how loud you are. It's about how **unignorable** you become.

You've spent the last six chapters learning the skills you need to do what most others couldn't imagine. You are set up to do the work most people avoid: getting clear, getting specific, building structure, and building trust. Now the time for quiet preparation is over. The time for action has come.

Don't wait for perfect conditions. Don't wait for consensus. Don't wait for someone else to take the first step.

You're the one who moves first.

You're the one who holds the line when it gets hard.

You're the one who makes sure this fight doesn't fade into the next shift or the next crisis.

8
Organizational Structure

"So never lose an opportunity of urging a practical beginning, however small, for it is wonderful how often in such matters the mustard-seed germinates and roots itself."
- Florence Nightingale

Essential Structure

When I started out, I didn't have a fancy team or a polished plan. I had conviction and enough education to be dangerous. That's where it begins. Not with a hashtag. Not with a committee. With the bones of an operation that tells the world: "I'm not going away."

At the most basic level, thriving activism requires five things. A mission, a leader, a team, an army, and, in most cases, funding.

Having a mission seems obvious, but I want to break this down because it's a trap that I see many organizations falling into. For some, they manage, while others go down in flames.

You must have an issue everyone can get behind, that is obvious and pretty easy. The hard part is **sticking to that mission** and not getting caught up and pulled in too many directions. Some describe what I am discussing as a "single issue group." Meaning that you only address the single issue at hand and not anything else.

For this book, the mission is to resuscitate nursing. All things resuscitating nursing can fall under your umbrella. Caution comes in when you start adding things not directly related to nursing. To be most effective on an issue involving people from all backgrounds, I strongly encourage you to leave the non-nursing problems out.

Even though you are involved in political activism, leave party politics out of it. Political backgrounds in nursing are diverse and fairly irrelevant. We are taught to leave our biases behind and care for the individual in front of us. That is precisely the kind of attitude we want to carry.

We must understand that we are up against industry giants formidable boogeymen in the form of the medical industrial complex, big pharma, the entire insurance industry, the US government, and giant hospital corporations. We do not have the luxury of alienating a whole group of people who agree with us on the issue we are fighting.

The same goes for religion; it's okay for your faith to be part of your why, but you need to be sure that you aren't projecting your faith on others so that it drives them from our mission- **resuscitating nursing**.

Certain nursing issues will draw a hard line of division between nurses, quickly dividing ranks based on many factors. If you choose to address abortion, gender dysphoria, vaccinations, alternative medicine, or any other number of hot-button nursing issues, be sure to consider how this can impact other avenues in advocacy.

I want to be clear, I am not discouraging you from advocating for your patients or taking action on an issue you are passionate about. I am simply suggesting that, due to the divisiveness of these topics, you consider how you want to approach and handle these issues before starting your organization.

The Strategic Triage Framework can help determine whether you want to make one of these hot-button issues your primary focus, wait to address them until more generalized nursing issues are resolved, or identify areas that you will not address as an organization. Once you have considered this, draw that line from the beginning and be consistent. This will build your credibility and ensure that there are no misgivings about what you are doing. It will reduce some drama within your army and even within your team.

Either way, remember you must have a clear and well-defined mission and boundaries for topics you aren't prepared to act on.

Knowing your limitations, you can be prepared to say, "I see how important it is. However, we only have the resources to focus here." You can also say, "Yes, I see how that is an issue; however, taking that fight is beyond our scope. You are welcome to start an organization to take up that fight."

We have discussed the team and your army at length, but I haven't provided them with specific definitions yet.

Your team comprises the various roles discussed in Chapter Five. These are the individuals who help keep the movement going; they may also be referred to as co-leaders, sub-leaders, or volunteers.

I have said it before and will say again, you (the leader) can't do this alone. You must have a team because, very quickly, you will come to realize that the weight of being a changemaker is considerable. We don't run codes alone. How could we possibly resuscitate nursing alone?

Next, the Army. You might wonder what the difference is between the team and the army. It's a subtle difference, but defining.

Your army is the group of people to whom you send your calls to action. They make phone calls and attend meetings, but are not leaders- they are simply followers. An army is imperative and may be segmented into different lists. The lists might come from different petitions or issues. Keeping track of who is joining your movement for what reasons can be helpful as you move forward.

Some will come on for one issue, and others will jump in to help with everything you do. These are all ok. Delineating them will be helpful when working on different topics or trying to increase pressure. You won't necessarily need to reach your entire army for all things. Tracking differences will be exceptionally helpful, so you don't burn people out or drive them away.

Your army is the most critical part of your movement. People, especially politicians, know this. They will want to get a hold of your list.

DO NOT LET THEM.

Your army and their contact information are a prized possession. Protect it like the bladder scanner!

Seriously. I am not kidding. Do not include the contact info when you release petitions to their intended audience. When I deliver petitions to legislators, I only include the first and last name and zip code.

As a side note, it is essential to deliver petitions; therefore, make sure to consider how you will do so. You can use tools like "mail merge" on Microsoft Word or "bulk upload" on Canva.

I want to pause for just a moment.

Following this advice, keeping that list private may be difficult for you, so I want to ensure you take that to heart. Consider why the contact information for your army would be valuable to politicians and other groups, even those with friendly intentions.

As soon as they have your list, they can replace you.

They can deliver their message directly to your army.

If a politician gets hold of your people's contact info, they will have a direct line to tell YOUR ARMY why you are wrong, talk them off the ledge, or maybe even threaten them. Friendly groups, even though you might be agreeing at the moment, they may take a different stance on an issue later down the road, and if you hand YOUR ARMY over to them, it could make mobilizing your army much more difficult in those fights.

Lastly, perhaps most importantly, you are morally obligated to protect these people's privacy. In this day and age, we are getting bombarded with spam and data breaches. If people trust you with their contact information, you had better protect it and ensure you act with integrity. One false move could cause you to lose your good standing, and that in and of itself could end your movement.

That brings us to our last area- funding. If people trust you, they have shared their contact information with you, which might help you fund your mission. Most people don't like to think about this aspect of things. However, it is necessary. If you are planning a small movement, making changes on your unit, or even at your small, privately owned hospital, you may not need funding. But, as soon as you start thinking about regional or statewide activism, you should begin fundraising because costs add up quickly. Therefore, you must understand how to generate revenue and sustain your movement's growth.

Funding

Honestly, if you are truly resuscitating nursing, you want to grow your moment, you want people to buy in. When people give, they're not just funding your fight. They're claiming it as their own. That sense of ownership will help your mission thrive.

In the next section, we will discuss the different organizational structures you might choose and how they will significantly impact how much time you will invest in fundraising.

For the most part, my experience tied to success comes from setting up a nonprofit, so most of the information from here on will be based on the idea that you are not just working from a social media page or a group messaging app. If you want real change, you need a real organization.

I don't say this to discourage those of you making changes within your unit or small, privately owned hospitals. Those areas are limited in scope, and your army will be on a much smaller scale, and you may find creative ways around fundraising. Resuscitating nursing will require changes in major hospital systems and government bureaucracy. Again, that doesn't mean you can't use these tactics. It just means you will have to adjust accordingly for your needs.

Even if you plan a small "concerted activity," you must talk with an attorney to see what your state requires. Some states have thresholds as low as $500 before you have to report. In the scheme of things, that isn't much at all. Whatever you do, you will want to ensure your movement keeps things squeaky clean and by the book.

If you follow the tactics in this book, you are confrontational. You will make enemies. When you start landing big punches and winning fights, they will look for the easiest way to stop you in your tracks- finances are typically the best way to do that. Financial mismanagement, even accidental, could cost you your credibility, your cause, and sometimes your personal finances or freedom. Don't risk this area; check in with an attorney.

Obviously, there are many ways to get out there and pull in money, but again, we want to ensure we are staying above board. Some of you might consider using one of your personal money-sharing apps like PayPal, Venmo, or Cash App. I would advise against these for a couple of reasons.

First of all, some of your teammates may find this a bit concerning initially, but certainly, if there is ever discord or success, you don't want to give anyone a reason to drag your name through the mud.

Secondly, from a practical standpoint, that money flows into your personal account, so you must keep impeccable documentation of where the money is coming from and where it is going. Again, your personal accounts could be under the microscope if something goes sideways. Who wants their personal accounts to be scrutinized? I would not risk this avenue.

Alternatively, you could use crowdfunding sources like "GiveSendGo" or "GoFundMe". I think most people are burned out on these, and they have started to feel spammy or scammy.

The plus side is that you don't need an official organization set up, but the money must be transferred into someone's account. You could even open a new checking account with the sole purpose of using it for your activism. This will provide you with precise tracking of the amount of money being transferred and when. You still have some risk that your personal accounts could be called into question, but it is a bit cleaner than using your own money apps, and there is slightly more credibility.

Don't groan… but bake sales, candy bars, and laundry soap are all options. They may be overdone and quite a bit of work. Still, it might not be a bad idea for a small group that needs to scrape together a few hundred dollars for some basics, especially if you have the time and an immediate financial need in your concerted activities.

The final stretch on fundraising will be based on my knowledge of founding and running a non-profit organization. If you plan to do the same, I would fail if I didn't tell you to **start fundraising immediately**.

Some pragmatic individuals may think, "Well, what if I raise too much money and don't need it?"

Realistically, this will not be a problem. The things we discuss in this chapter and the next, "Infrastructure," cost money.

Printing, money.
Emails, money.
Text messages, money.

Website, money.
Gas & lodging, money.
Setting up a nonprofit, money.

Back to your question, "What if I raise too much money and don't need it?" Simple- you donate it to an organization similar to yours. In the worst-case scenario, if you need suggestions, please don't hesitate to contact me. I will help you find an organization with values or locations comparable to yours, ensuring that your donor's money is not wasted.

Again, realistically, you will not raise "too much." If your organization is thriving and growing, you will need the funding to continue your mission or take on bigger projects. I speak from experience.

One of the single best decisions I made when I started my organization was setting up an official donation site with recurring monthly donors.

At the moment, an issue is new and hot, or you are in the midst of a big battle, fundraising will never be easier.

BE READY.

Fundraising is hard, I get it. No one likes to ask for money, but if you want to be effective, and I know you do, you have to be able to fund your movement. No one else is going to step in and do it for you. You may find someone who doesn't loathe it at some point, but those opportunities are rare. If you find someone with work experience in fundraising and who enjoys it, latch on to them and never let go! They are rare gems.

Even less likely than finding a dedicated and enthusiastic fundraiser is finding a wealthy benefactor who will slap thousands of dollars down on the table.

The truth is that it just doesn't happen. Large donors can and do come along, but Individuals with large amounts of expendable income want to see results before they invest. It will only be after significant wins and persistence.

There is no better place to start with your persistence than fundraising, because small amounts add up over time and are typically what funds movements. In the next chapter, we will discuss various fundraising platform options and provide tips to help you sort through the noise of which platform to use.

After all, struggling with these things keeps you from doing the work and expanding your movement. Believe me, if you apply the tactics outlined in this book, you will be effective and grow.

Before starting serious fundraising, you must set down a strong foundation with an organizational structure, which can be intimidating and confusing. In the next section, I will do my best to give you a mini-course based on the available options.

Starting with a Strong Foundation

I was so incredibly blessed by that first political class I took. Not only did it teach me the basics and give me permission to act with integrity rather than engage in political games, but it also gave me a fantastic mentor.

I would have had no clue how to get started or where to go. I probably would have fallen flat on my face and not formed a 501(c)4. I certainly wouldn't have taken fundraising seriously. I will do my best to give you that same foundation in this accessible book rather than an 8-hour, face-to-face, party-centric, drink from the fire hose of politics course.

There are numerous ways to build an organization, but only a handful that make sense for the type of work we're doing. These structures can provide your mission with the legal backing, protection, and strategic flexibility necessary for growth. Each serves a different purpose, and one will likely stand out depending on your goals.

Let's take a quick look at the most relevant options for nurse-led advocacy, in no particular order:

- **501(c)(3)** – *Charitable Nonprofit:* Best for public education, scholarships, and non-political initiatives. Donations are tax-deductible, but political activity is heavily restricted.
- **501(c)(4)** – *Social Welfare Organization:* Designed for advocacy and grassroots mobilization. You can lobby freely and even discuss political campaigns while being tax-exempt. Donations are not tax-deductible, but the impact is enormous.
- **501(c)(6)** – *Professional Association or Business League:* Created to promote the common interests of a profession, perfect for advancing nursing standards, hosting conferences, or offering member benefits. Lobbying is permitted, but the focus must remain on member interests.
- **LLC (Limited Liability Company)** – A flexible, for-profit *business* structure for those offering consulting, coaching, or education services. It allows complete control and protects personal assets, but limits political activity and doesn't accept donations.
- **Union** – A formal collective bargaining unit that negotiates contracts, defends worker rights, and offers legal protections. Strong but slow-moving and often bureaucratic.
- **Concerted Activity** – Protected under the National Labor Relations Act (NLRA), this refers to informal collective actions by workers (like group complaints or refusals to work under unsafe conditions). No formal organization is required, but it offers some legal protection for speaking out.
- **Private Mutual Aid** – *Support group* ideal for sharing resources, protecting one another from retaliation, and creating informal solidarity. It is not a legal entity, but it is excellent for building trust and support when risk is high.

By now, you certainly have an idea of the battles you are facing and which way you are headed, and you have committed to the tactics in this book. So, we will further frame what those tactics look like with each option above.

501(c)(3) – Charitable Nonprofit

A 501(c)(3) is what most people think of when they hear the word “nonprofit.” These charitable organizations focus on education, public service, and community benefit. Consider this the right option if your primary goal is to educate the public, offer scholarships, establish a foundation, or host programs such as nurse training, community workshops, or health awareness campaigns. It’s especially effective if you’re trying to reach the public, build trust, or apply for grants.

One of the most significant advantages of a 501(c)(3) is that donations are **tax-deductible** and **tax-exempt**. This can attract donors, foundations, and corporate sponsors who are more comfortable giving to an organization with this designation. It’s also the most “respected” in traditional nonprofit spaces because they are largely apolitical.

> ***Pro-Tip:*** It is crucial to understand the difference between tax-deductible and tax-exempt. Tax-exempt status means that by following the government’s rules, your organization is not required to pay federal income tax. Tax-deductible does not relate to your tax status, but the ability of donors to “write off” donations on their taxes.

However, the downside is *significant* when it comes to advocacy.

If you create a 501(c)(3), you will be heavily restricted when it comes to lobbying or any political activity. You will **NOT** be able to use the tactics outlined in this book. If you do, even accidentally, you will face severe fines and jeopardize your status.

You might wonder, “What can I do with a 501(c)3?”

You can “educate” lawmakers, but you can’t push legislation.

You can “raise awareness,” but you can’t name and call out bad political actors or get involved in elections.

If you're trying to create *real* change and not just talk about it, you'll quickly feel boxed in by your 501(c)3. This structure works great for general education or community support, but if your goal is policy reform or holding leadership accountable, it will not be enough on its own.

**Keep your eyes peeled for a crash course on wtajourney.com/rnbook for information on utilizing a 501(c)3 alongside other organization types.

501(c)(4) – Social Welfare Organization

This is where the gloves come off, and you can start cooking with fire. A 501(c)(4) is built for advocacy and the tactics outlined in this book.

It's a nonprofit, which gives credibility, but it exists specifically **to promote social welfare**, including **lobbying, mobilizing, and political action**. If your vision includes writing legislation, pressuring policymakers, organizing campaigns, or getting involved in elections, this is the tool for the job.

The major pro? **Freedom**. A 501(c)(4) can name names, organize rallies, publish voter guides, and unapologetically apply pressure. It's designed to stir the pot. You don't have to play political games. You have a mission, and this structure protects your ability to fight for it. If you're forming an army of nurses and patients to take on corrupt institutions or expose weak leadership, this is your battlefield basecamp.

You do still have some restrictions and guidelines to maintain your tax-exempt status. Namely, ensuring that you are not participating in campaign activity. Specifically, the use of words like endorse, support, or oppose.

Some 501(c) 4 organizations will engage in this behavior. They are playing a risky game. The vague IRS rules state that campaign involvement may not be the organization's primary activity. It is generally accepted that political campaign activities must be less than 49% of the organization's activities.

Organizations participating in political campaign activities may be subject to federal tax per section 527(f) of the Internal Revenue Code if they join in endorsing, supporting, or opposing candidates.

However, 501(c) 4 organizations can participate in *informing* voters by conducting issue discussions. This topic will be addressed more thoroughly in the Resuscitating Nursing Mentorship program. These basics will certainly help. Just remember, this is not legal advice, and any questions should be addressed with your attorney.[1]

The downside is that donations to a 501(c)(4) are **not tax-deductible,** which can turn some larger donors off or limit the amount they are willing to give without the incentive of a tax write-off. You also won't qualify for most grants. But in my experience, the kind of people who give to a 501(c)(4) aren't doing it for a tax write-off. They're doing it because they believe in the mission. And if your messaging is strong, those people will come. You must give them something to rally around.

I am biased because this has worked well for me in other advocacy endeavors. Still, for the kind of change it will take to resuscitate nursing, 501(c)4's give you the non-profit credibility and tax-exemption without sacrificing your ability to call out bad political actors.

---

1 Internal Revenue Service. (n.d.). *Political activity and social welfare.* U.S. Department of the Treasury. Retrieved May 26, 2025, from https://www.irs.gov/charities-non-profits/other-non-profits/political-activity-and-social-welfare

Internal Revenue Service. (n.d.). *Social welfare organizations.* U.S. Department of the Treasury. Retrieved May 26, 2025, from https://www.irs.gov/charities-non-profits/other-non-profits/social-welfare-organizations

501(c)(6) – Professional Association or Business League

This is the go-to option if your mission is to elevate the profession of nursing itself. A 501(c)(6) is often used for trade associations and business leagues, think chambers of commerce, or in our case, **nursing associations**. This structure is designed to protect and promote the members of a profession, not the public. It's ideal if you want to focus on advancing nursing standards, providing continuing education, hosting conferences, publishing research, or lobbying on behalf of licensed professionals.

What makes 501(c)(6) attractive is its ability to **lobby without restriction**. Unlike a 501(c)(3), there are no caps on political advocacy, and unlike a 501(c)(4), it doesn't require you to frame your mission around the public. It's about **you and your members**. That makes it powerful for internal reforms: credentialing, policy changes, licensure standards, and direct pressure on hospital systems or state boards.

The limitation? It's member-focused by law. That means if your mission extends to protecting patients, or **if you're trying to reach the public or raise funds from outside supporters, this may not be the best fit on its own**. This may hinder your ability to fundraise and expand considerably. You also won't be eligible for most traditional grants or public fundraising campaigns. My guess is that, as a change maker, you want to do more than organize nurses across institutions and build a politically active professional association.

The 501(c)(6) might be a supplemental support group to utilize after a well-established 501(c)4 is in place and has a strong organizational foundation.

LLC – Limited Liability Company

An LLC is a for-profit business structure, but don't let that scare you off. An LLC can be a powerful tool for nurses, offering consulting, educational services, advocacy workshops, and even legal nurse consulting. It gives you complete control, shields your personal assets, and allows you to turn your work into a sustainable income stream that can help fund your advocacy.

The strength of an LLC is **flexibility**. You can sell courses, charge for speaking engagements, create downloadable guides, and run your platform like a business, all while keeping your mission front and center. If you're building a personal brand around nurse advocacy, leadership development, or reform education, this may be the best way to structure it.

But it's not right for everything. You can't accept donations, you won't get grant funding, and you'll be limited in the type of political action you can take directly under the business name.

You can, however, use the revenue from your LLC to support a separate nonprofit or political group. Some leaders may use this model as a hybrid, earning money through one vehicle and funding their movement through another. However, you must ensure you have an attorney who is well-versed in these topics.

In my opinion, creating an LLC is risky, primarily if you are employed by an entity that you might be targeting, which could create a significant conflict of interest. Additional legal issues may crop up, too.

Union

Unions are the most formalized, and often believed to be the most powerful, way to organize collective action in the workplace. A union exists to negotiate contracts, protect employee rights, and engage in formal grievance procedures. If your hospital is hemorrhaging nurses and no one is listening, a union can force them to the table and legally require changes.

If everything goes right and you get a "good union," the upside is enormous. With enough support, unions can secure better pay, enforce safe staffing, and shield whistleblowers from retaliation. They also have access to legal teams, strike funds, and formal protections under labor law. Unions can seem like a lifeline for significant, systemic issues inside institutions.

When creating a union, you'll also need to **meet specific legal requirements** to form or join one, and that process isn't fast.

And they come with baggage.

Unions are slow-moving, often highly bureaucratic, and not always responsive to grassroots needs. Depending on the union's bylaws and conditions, you may be required to strike and lose your ability to negotiate with hospital leadership directly. Worst of all, **State or National leadership may have different priorities than the nurses on the ground**. They may even refuse to represent your ideas or take up initiatives you bring to them.

Your union could quickly become an additional hoop you must jump through to solicit change. If that change opposes the union's goals, then you may be in a world of trouble.

You might wonder how we can take action in a hospital setting without facing retaliation if we don't have a union. The following section addresses this, but remember, there are never guarantees, even with a union; your job is not guaranteed. Further, when you get good at taking on these battles, you will become a target, which might mean losing your job.

Concerted Activity

This is one of the most basic forms of activism because it doesn't require forming any organization. **Concerted Activity** is protected under the National Labor Relations Act (NLRA), giving you the legal right to speak up, protest unsafe conditions, or take collective action with other employees, even if you're not in a union.

Concerted Activity gives time to initiate activism before you can start an organization.

What does this look like? Two or more nurses refusing to take on dangerous assignments, jointly signing letters, or documenting concerns about working conditions as a group. Most actions are protected as long as they are **collective and aimed at improving working conditions.** The National Labor Relations Board (NLRB) states point blank, "Your employer cannot discharge, discipline, or threaten you for, or coercively question you about, this 'protected concerted' activity." That is pretty powerful.

The trick is **knowing your rights** and when to call for help. You may still want to double-check with an employment attorney to verify your limitations.

> ***Pro Tip:*** You may see discussions about organized walkouts as part of these protected activities. I would like to emphasize that as a nurse, you cannot abandon your patients. Once you take the assignment, you are responsible for those patients. Before organizing a mid-shift walkout, ensure you understand the potential legal ramifications. They may not come from the hospital themselves. If something happens to a patient during a walkout, you may face a civil lawsuit, and we know that your hospital won't hesitate to throw you under the bus.

The risk is that most employers don't like it and may retaliate anyway. But if they do, and you've documented everything, you may have a strong case with the National Labor Relations Board.

Concerted activity is the fastest, cheapest, and most immediate form of pressure nurses can use when conditions are unsafe and formal internal processes have failed.

It's not a long-term structure, but it is a legal right, and you should know how to use it to avoid delays in your activism. Unfortunately, many nurses with good intentions freeze out of fear of retribution. Knowing about your rights under concerted activity can help eliminate that.[2]

> ***Pro Tip:*** When engaging with the NLRB, they may send representatives to discuss options for a formal union. While these come with perceived benefits, unionizing brings in an additional layer of politicians you must deal with.

Private Mutual Aid or Peer-Support Network

A **mutual aid or peer-support network** is a group of nurses who agree to support one another in times of need. That might look like sharing resources, offering emotional support, collecting donations for someone who's been retaliated against, or quietly helping each other document unethical conditions.

You probably have this on a small scale in your unit, and it may start to creep out into other areas, especially when safety risks are present and trust in the system is low. You don't need to file paperwork, pay fees, or build a website. You need people who are committed to protecting each other. Think of it as a nurse-led underground where you and your team develop bonds and hold each other together amid desperation.

Of course, the drawback is that it offers **no legal protection or formal authority**. It's not a nonprofit, a union, or a business. It won't even get you a seat at the table, but it might keep your team alive long enough to build something that does. This model is handy early on, or in hostile environments where exposure could lead to retaliation. It's the heart of grassroots organizing; people watching each other's backs until the movement is strong enough to stand in the open.

2 National Labor Relations Board. (n.d.). *Concerted activity*. U.S. Government. Retrieved May 26, 2025, from https://www.nlrb.gov/about-nlrb/rights-we-protect/the-law/employees/concerted-activity-0

Putting the Pieces Together

You don't need to have every detail figured out before you begin, but you do need to build on solid ground. Organizational structure isn't just about paperwork. It's about protecting your people, amplifying your mission, and ensuring you don't get burnt out or get buried in red tape before you even start. The proper structure gives your movement staying power, and the wrong one can sabotage it before it takes its first breath.

For the kind of work it will take to *resuscitate nursing*, to challenge bad laws, call out corrupt leadership, and defend both nurses and patients in a system that often fails them, there is no better tool than the 501(c)(4). It gives you room to act boldly and unapologetically. It gives you a home base for mobilization and a banner your supporters can rally behind. If you're ready to go beyond complaints and lead meaningful, public change, this is how you do it.

Just remember: organizational structure doesn't have to be perfect. **It has to be purposeful.** Pick the structure that gives you the reach, protection, and authority you need, and build it strong enough to carry the weight of what's coming next.

Because we're not just fighting for better conditions, we're fighting for the soul of this profession. And we're not here to play nice. We're here to resuscitate nursing.

What good is an organization if no one knows about it or where to find information?

Nothing.

If people don't know who you are, what you stand for, and have no way to investigate other than talking to you, they won't be interested. Nurses are cautious and want to ensure that they aren't taking unnecessary risks or causing more problems for themselves. Let's face it. We are all exhausted trying to hold the wheels on this bus.

You need a quick and accessible way for your organization to be introduced and a means of communication. That is precisely what we will dive into in the next chapter!

9
Infrastructure
How to Scale, Sustain, and Protect the Movement

"Let us never consider ourselves finished nurses... we must be learning all of our lives."
- Florence Nightingale

Infrastructure isn't glamorous, but it separates movements that fizzle out from those that make history.

The last thing I want to talk about is infrastructure. It's boring, a bit tedious, and there are numerous decisions and options. I tend to struggle with analysis paralysis because I want the perfect tool.

I also don't want to give "bad advice," and I am not sure there is a perfect recommendation with so many products out there. These decisions have always been challenging for me, which is why this is the last chapter. I will reference a few of my favorite products, primarily those that work well for me, but I encourage you to explore and find what's right for you. Of course, if you find something amazing, please let me know. After all, the purpose of this is to give you the tools and information you need so you can resuscitate nursing!

Ok, here we go… Infrastructure is essential; without it, your movement will likely be nothing more than a flash in the pan. We will discuss mobilization tools, websites, fundraising, and more.

Website

When I started my journey in activism, I got to work founding the 501(c) (4) and jumped straight into creating a website.

Why?

Once you've nailed down your structure, it's time to build your base of operations. A website isn't optional. It's your headquarters. It conveys to people that you're serious, organized, and not going anywhere. This is where you control the message, rally your army, expose the truth, and direct the next move. Whether collecting signatures, publishing receipts, or calling people to action, your website is where the mission lives.

Pointing people to a professional and well-organized website is essential to be taken seriously, not only by donors, but by the media and politicians you are fighting against.

Think of it as "sizing up" the threat. Politicians will strut over and investigate. They will look down their noses and "see" what you have…

"Oh, they have a small group of nurses, ok. Not a big deal. This will blow over soon."

"They have a social media page, that's cute. I will use that against them. I can pull screenshots, and if someone says something inappropriate, I can use it to break their ranks or even shut the whole thing down."

"Oh, they have filed for a 501(c)--, and they have a website… (Pause with more scrutiny) They can communicate. (Gasp) They are protecting themselves and know their rights… (grunt) We might have a problem here. I'd better take this seriously."

That legitimacy gains necessary traction and helps build your army.

While politicians and adversaries are disappointed to see that you have a quality website, your potential allies will rejoice. They can use your website as their central hub of information. Review your mission, find out how serious you are, and determine if they are willing to put their neck out on the line next to yours.

Be sure to set yourself apart from other organizations. Accentuate your strengths, goals, and beliefs that answer the PROBLEM that your nurses are facing. Avoid language that may come off as condescending. Just stick to objective facts.

Simply by identifying the issues and *offering solutions*, you are light years ahead of most, if not all, others. This builds trust and credibility. It also shows those around you that you mean business.

You are not waiting around for someone else to find the solution.
You aren't going to be standing around complaining.
You are a change maker.
You are resuscitating nursing.

People don't want to waste their time tracking down information, hunting for talking points, or figuring out how to share the message with their circles. This is where your website comes in.

Rather than search through random emails, social media, or Google Docs, they can go to your website and find exactly what they need. Plus, you don't have to worry about losing all your work if your social media site gets shut down or your profile gets hacked. Your website will still be standing. Even more importantly, your website is accessible to those who don't utilize social media.

If your people struggle to get information, they will struggle to mobilize.

Mobilization is a key use of my website. I use it to publish handy worksheets, house my petitions, share information about events, and, most importantly, keep a blog running that provides all the details I can't fit into a text or email. The blog also serves as a living testimony to the actions and success of the organization.

Showing success and effective mobilization will be key if you intend to garner donations. Again, if they have to hunt for it, they won't do it. My website features a dedicated page for donations, and I incorporate subtle cues to encourage donations throughout the site. I also have a floating tab on the side so the viewer constantly has this in their periphery.

During legislative season, when things move at the speed of light and there are important dates to remember, I love adding calendars so that my members are aware of deadlines. This is imperative to maximizing your time.

Equipping your website with education and ensuring transparency are key features. Running an organization is busy. If you are the only source of information or education, your time will run out FAST. You will spend hours repeating yourself to well-meaning volunteers who never seem to get anything done.

Why?

At least initially, they depend on you to know and understand where to go. Empowering your team and army through education on your website is a time-saver that every leader should utilize.

Speaking of time-saving, when you collect signatures and contact information on paper, transferring them to electronic means takes time. Not many people like data entry; even worse, we all make errors. One wrong letter in an email or one incorrect digit in a phone number, and you will not reach your target. Building petitions right through your website is a great way to save time and money. Another overlooked benefit is organization- you don't have to worry about yet another password to remember.

Many people think that you need specific software or tools for petition development. You don't. You can even start without a website using Google Forms or similar services. But I do it all right from my website.

I use text and simple contact forms built into my drag-and-drop website. They transform the data into a spreadsheet I can use for mail merges in Word or bulk uploads in Canva. Using these spreadsheets to update your contacts for emails or texting is super simple.

Don't let your petitions be a simple endpoint. Make sure you incorporate an additional action. Sometimes, that is a simple downloadable graphic for sharing. For others, it is an invitation to a meeting or a private social media page.

Many websites have a "redirect" upon submission of contact forms. That means once they submit their information, they can be shown a message or sent to a website. That's where I create a page that thanks the signer for taking action and includes an embedded donation form. Hot petitions can be surprisingly great fundraisers! Do not miss this opportunity.

After my petition is launched, I keep updating that page. I add details and updates below the petition so that people can review our actions and progress. It serves both as a means of growing and informing my army. As I recirculate the webpage, people who have already signed it stay up-to-date, and those just learning about the issue can sign the petition, continuing to grow the movement.

> ***Pro Tip:*** When setting up petitions, use the same order for each new petition. I require Name, email, and zip code on everything, but I add phone and a comment as optional. I encourage you to keep the same order across different petitions or forms because this will make it easier when combining lists for a "master document." Comments by the signer can serve as additions to the printed petitions or as encouragement for you. Sometimes I even use them on quotes as memes to promote the petition.

Education can also translate to posting the receipts or "wall of shame." This is a designated area where you and your team strategically post the failed promises of the politicians you are facing. Most likely, this will be something that builds over time and can show the story of failure in the politician's own words.

At the same time, you are using your website as a political sword. It is also a shield that provides protection.

Your website contains your polished message and tells your story the way you want it to be told. You do not need to rely on media interviews for soundbites or items to share. You create your own press by mobilizing your people so they direct others to your message. This eliminates the need for potentially damaging interviews with the media, which are often aimed at creating controversy or tarnishing your reputation. It also keeps your message on point and prevents it from drifting.

If you are hit with a smear campaign, you can point right back to your website easily, declaring what you stand for and why.

Truthfully, most of the time you won't need to respond to bad press. If people ask, point them back to the website, but don't go out of your way to address bad press or attacks. Most of the time, these events are not as big as they feel. When you respond in a 'large" way, you inform your army of something they otherwise might not have heard about.

If you respond to bad press, do so in a way that focuses on your strengths, values, and track record that refutes the attack without mentioning it. You can do this easily through the blog. Those who have heard about the controversy will look for answers. Others will see an excellent piece you did, claiming your stance and broadcasting your solutions.

Now that you know more about the importance and function of your website, we can further explore its structure. They can vary widely based on your skills and goals.

Anymore, websites are so easy to develop and publish, especially with platforms like Canva and others that allow you to have a one-page website put together in minutes. You can also easily use drag-and-drop sites like Wix or Weebly. They both have had their own benefits, and I do enjoy using them. However, Wix is more modern with many add-on features that you can tailor to your specific needs. Overall, the platform is pretty user-friendly and can be rapidly edited.

Your forward-facing website needs to be foolproof and easy to navigate. If people have to navigate through a series of different pages to reach their destination, they will struggle and likely leave. Setting up a basic organization will be imperative.

Start with a home page explaining your mission, a short, relatable introduction explaining who and why you are, and a contact form where people can sign up for updates or communications. I added one of these to each page of my website.

Next, you can move into the ACTION mode. This can be titled anything you want, but remember, simple is good. "Action" or "petitions" are perfect headings. I have a main page listing petitions. Then they can click each petition they want to sign. Having two or three petitions helps me determine which issues are hot buttons. I am always careful not to have too many at once, though. You want to keep your mission strong and on point.

Some people will go through and sign all the petitions, and others will sign a single issue. These nuances help refine my messaging and sometimes help me determine which direction to go in the following year.

Whenever I conduct a petition, I always offer my signers a way to financially support the cause. Do not miss out on this prime opportunity. The individuals signing the petition believe in your mission. They are willing to give you their contact information. As soon as they hit the submit button, they should see "Thank you for signing the [petition name], we can't do this without you. Please donate to support the cause." In more or less words.

I like to embed my donation forms. We will talk about how to do that in the next section. But before we move on to that, remember you can structure your website to fit your needs, including the blog we discussed earlier, an introduction to board members, volunteer positions, sign-ups, media kits, education, and so much more.

This is your forward-facing representation. Make it user-friendly and tailored to your issue, and always give them the opportunity to donate.

Donation Platforms

As discussed earlier, fundraising is a big deal.

No one likes to hear that, but it doesn't make it any less accurate. If you are creating an organization that will make history, you must fundraise.

You are not taking people's money; you are putting it to good use for a cause they believe in. So let's make this uncomfortable idea of fundraising a little less painful.

In this section, I will walk you through the keywords and fees associated with fundraising, so you feel more confident in making a decision.

There are numerous platforms available, and I have experience with a few. I will only review my favorite. Most platforms offer recurring donations, making it easy for individuals to sign up and manage their donations through the platform. They also offer a wide range of other services, and I have found it easy to embed these donation forms directly into my website by simply copying and pasting the link they provide.

It can be overwhelming when you start looking at different options and see all the fees, or worse, don't see the fees. When you work hard for a cause and put in the effort to fundraise, you don't want that money to seemingly disappear before it even goes to your cause. The following will help you make those decisions quickly and avoid analysis paralysis due to a fear of making mistakes or having difficulty understanding the differences between platforms.

Basic terms you need to know:

Processing fee: This fee is charged when using a credit card or mobile payment method. Whenever a credit card is processed, the banking institution must verify that the funds are available and notify the cardholder of the debit, etc. So, there is a fee for this service. This is commonly done through a company like Stripe or PayPal. I have noticed that PayPal is more expensive than Stripe. These fees range between 2.2% and 5.0% PLUS an additional $0.30 - $0.75 per transaction.

Platform fee: This fee is charged by the "platform" or website used to collect the information and provide you with easily embedded forms, data, analytics, etc. This fee covers the platform's organizational services, which have simplified the process. Stripe is not nearly as user-friendly as some of the donation platforms. Platform fees range between 1.5% and 5%.

Subscription-free: This is a fee you pay simply for accessing tools on a platform and may be present with both of the other fees! They may have a sliding scale based on the number of contacts you have. Watch for "*Starting at" to indicate that costs will increase rapidly.

My head was spinning when I read about the various fees, and I struggled to decide which platform was the best. Another limiting factor for me was that I wasn't starting with any money, so I had to make a decision quickly, and subscription fees were not an option.

Ultimately, I chose donorbox.org. It was reputable and had a lot of features, and I could get started without any money, i.e., no subscription fee. The fees for processing and platform seemed to be the lowest combined in the market. Additionally, they allow you to ask your donors to cover them and don't add any extra costs. So when starting small yet wanting something comprehensive, Donorbox was the way to go for me.

Donorbox offers a paid premium plan, which I have not utilized. Periodically, I review the platform options to determine what makes sense from a budgetary perspective. Over five years later, my organization has remained with donorbox.org.

I recently began seeing reels for a company called Zeffy.com and thought that a free platform that promises not to sell your info might be a great option until I started digging a little deeper under the surface. While Zeffy.com is free, the "tips" or donor-covered fees are listed at 17% of the donation. This absolutely blew my mind. I could not believe they would ask donors to make that kind of "tip". I certainly didn't feel comfortable with it, so it was an automatic no.

The platform may be alluring for some because the fees are 0%... Until you read the fine print. Personally, I would rather have that extra 17% directed back to my organization. Using Donorbox, I still have the option to ask donors to cover the fees. When they do, there is a minimal reduction in total donation. For example, at the time of this writing, if someone donates $10.70 (a $10 donation with a $0.70 fee), my organization gets $9.90.

That is fantastic!

I won't belabor the point here. There are many options, but Donorbox has been my preferred and has the most reasonable costs for what you get. I would encourage you to make a chart including the platform's name, fee schedules, pros and cons, and then pick the best for your organization. You should prioritize the easy transfer of donations into your bank account, as well as being able to track donations and fees for your accounting. **If this information is not easily accessible and transparent, I would be concerned.**

Being able to easily communicate and understand what is happening with your fundraising platform is just as important as how you communicate with your army.

While having a sound website and donation platform is imperative, it is essential to remember that that isn't the entire equation. You must communicate and engage directly with your army. Unless something is directly in their face, they aren't going to see it. So you need to be able to communicate directly with them. In the next portion of this chapter, we will discuss email, social media, and text messaging as a means of communication.

Direct Communication

In the initial phases, you might think that using your personal email and phone will be enough, but as I mentioned earlier, when you follow the tactics outlined in this book and build a movement, you will soon realize this is not the case. You will need a quick and easy way to get your message to the masses joining your army.

Just a quick tip- when you are starting out, and before you move into an email program, do yourself a favor. Do *not* use work emails. I'll say it again.

Do not use work emails.

Whether you realize it or not, your employer can and will go through your emails. They will use them against you, or worse, cut you off from access. If your entire army is wrapped up using work email, it can be gone in a heartbeat. Additionally, they can read and follow up with all your plans if they are communicated through those servers. Do not let this rookie mistake take your mission down before it even gets off the ground.

Email

Start a separate Gmail account, or use your preferred browser. Keep it clean and ensure that you check it regularly. If your website platform offers email with your URL name, that is your best bet. If you don't know what that means, it's your website name after the @, for example, info@yourwebsite.com.

You can use forwarders to ensure that it arrives in a personal email if the website email is difficult to access. A URL-based email address is required for some email platforms, so it's worth having set up early.

If you expect your organization to grow over 50-100 participants, you will need to consider an email service. Typically, standard accounts that send over 50 emails at once get flagged as spam. Like with everything else, there are loads of platforms out there. This was probably one of the most overwhelming decisions for me. I feel like all the plans are different and challenging to compare. When I started my organization, I had NO money. I was looking for cheap or free, and I knew I would eventually need to scale up.

Keeping something simple and relatively inexpensive was key. I was not too excited about writing emails. I don't read my own, and I think, as a whole, people's inboxes are flooded with trash every day. The motivation to keep up with it for little to no return was not motivating. Even after I started sending more emails, the data analytics only showed a read rate of 20-35%, which to me doesn't seem very practical.

Yet some people love them, and it is a standard practice, plus, even if they see your organization's name scroll through their inbox, it keeps you in their mind. The bottom line is that email is a necessity, but investing significantly is not a priority.

Just like with everything else, every couple of years I evaluate the programs I am using, if they are working, are cost-effective, and the best bang for my buck. And again, five years into activism, I am sticking with the email carrier I chose initially.

I currently use Brevo, and my most significant selling point was that they didn't charge me based on the number of contacts I had. The limitation of the free plan is the number of emails you can send daily, which was easy to work around at the time.

This is phenomenal for budding organizations, and the paid plans with Brevo are great and cheaper than most. Cost wasn't the only factor. I find the system really easy to use. Importing contacts is intuitive, and the email builder is all drag and drop. They have email templates, which you can make your own or use previous emails as templates.

They also do a great job of providing analytics for link clicks, etc. The platform offers Customer Relationship Management (CRM), texting, and other benefits. I honestly have not used the texting platform because the one I use is so much cheaper and has many amazing features.

I always send emails for calls to action, blog updates, meeting notices, and follow-ups. While email has near-instant delivery of thousands at a time, the read rate is poor and slow. I send texts when I have messages that I need to get out fast and want a high read rate!

Texting

Texting is probably my favorite thing to talk about! It is not because I enjoy it, but because it is very effective at reaching people quickly and growing your list!

This was one of the single best choices I made when starting in activism. I could easily go to a rally, hold a sign, or incorporate my texting number into a presentation or speech. I constantly share the number and put it on every graphic I send. I do each of these things to this day.

I added nearly 300 people to my list at a single rally and didn't have to enter their data manually. They all opted in by texting me. That saved me an incredible amount of time with data entry.

Most services offer keywords that allow you to send a custom message to those people and tag them based on what they text you. For example, I was at an Indiana University event, so I had the crowd text me "IU". Then, they received a predetermined message that I set up with links specific to my speech that day. Then, moving forward, I knew those people came in at IU.

During legislative season, I might use the keyword "Ratio" if we were fighting for better patient ratios. The service would automatically send back the message I attach to it, likely including the name and number of the politician they need to call. Again, I would then know who all participated in the call to action or event, and I can send future messages specifically to that group of people. I can also tell how engaged people are based on the number of keywords they have used! It is truly a fantastic tool. As with everything, not all systems are the same.

I use Project Broadcast, and the features and flow are absolutely fantastic. You get a dedicated phone number. This allows you to communicate directly with your army both as a group and on an individual basis.

Another benefit is that people can save your number in their contacts, ensuring they never confuse you with spam. Many other services have you use their short code or texts come from rotating numbers, which can be problematic for the reasons above.

Project broadcast offers multiple features. Some of my favorites are the call forwarding, keywords, and the additional fields for contact information.

Call forwarding is simple; it just means when a call comes into your Project Broadcast number, it is forwarded to your personal number, and no one is the wiser.

Many services offer keywords but typically only allow a certain number or charge for them in tiers. Project Broadcast offers an unlimited number, which is incredibly helpful because campaigns often run over the course of several years. This is especially true of educational campaigns, where individuals can gain knowledge or access resources by texting a specific keyword. It is terrific because automation takes care of it, and you don't have to worry about responding or taking any action.

The option of adding additional fields for contact information is also incredible. This allows me to, again, automate, collecting information like email, zip code, and so much more. Better yet, it can all be exported into a spreadsheet to upload to your email program or whatever else you use to communicate with your people.

But the absolute best part of the texts is the rapid-fire mobilization. I can text thousands of people with the click of a few buttons. During legislative season, when time is of the essence, this pays dividends.

I can schedule a text in minutes if I have the content. Typically, I can whip up a text quickly. I have also taught multiple other organizations how to successfully use it for rapid communication, improving connection with their army, and of course, fundraising.

I love watching the organizations I am mentoring tap into this tool and start growing. Being able to support that kind of growth is such a gift. I will continue offering crash courses about the Project Broadcast because the service is outstanding. You can find it on my website wtajourney.com/rnbook. Consider using my referral code; if you do, the crash course is yours for free. Just email me once you're signed up.

Text messaging through a service like this is a tremendous upgrade over old-school texting chains that can break down or are subject to a change in message. Further, when using these outdated techniques, you must trust portions of your army with many different people or send hundreds of texts through your phone. While you might have an unlimited texting plan, that does not stop you from getting texts at random times of the day… or night. It invades your privacy and makes it very hard to transfer if you need to step away, and someone else has to take over the organization.

Giving out your personal number could have a lot of negative ramifications, so at a minimum, using something like a Google Voice number to start would be advised. The great thing is that a Google Voice number is free. You add an app on your phone, and you can turn notifications off or transfer the number to another leader while you are on vacation or if you need to step away.

Overall, texting is the way to go. It keeps things clean, easy, and pretty automated. There will be some people who do not want texts. That is okay. I would encourage an accompanying email to reach them, and even a little social media to circulate things, and hopefully, grow your group.

Before we close out this chapter, let's go ahead and talk about social media.

Social Media

This can be a concern due to algorithms and censorship. Depending on your activism's style and level of controversy, you could quickly have your page taken down or even get banned. It is not uncommon for algorithms to limit your viewership or even throttle down your posts' reach. It is ridiculous but entirely possible, depending on the political climate.

I engage in social media that is convenient for me. I don't go out of my way to join every newly released platform. Usually, I won't join any of them. Some activists will be a little irritated by this. I politely let them know that spending time posting to different platforms is not the best use of my time, and I encouraged them to share our message on the platform through their pages. I always tell people they cannot create a page for my organization, but they can share our calls to action and point people back to our website and blog.

I encourage you to think about your audience and where they are. It seems like Facebook is a "more mature" crowd at the time of this writing; people here are typically 35+. If you want the younger crowd, Instagram, TikTok, or even X.com might be a better fit. You will likely find a more politically conservative crowd on X.com than on other sites. You will need to research and find out where your people are.

I am not a fan of social media and generally avoid it like the plague. I try to post because people have come to expect organizations to participate. However, trying to keep up with the rapid-fire changes and posting on multiple platforms can be overwhelming.

If I didn't have a tool that could post across all platforms, then I probably wouldn't post at all. It is just not a priority for me. I run a tight ship with our social media and don't particularly like getting off topic. I also have witnessed how one rogue volunteer can ruin an organization's reputation with the wrong tone or approach to sensitive issues. Delegating this task may be a bit of a risk. So, I screen these volunteers quite well, give parameters, and have them run things by me for a while before they post independently.

As much as I despise social media, it is a powerful tool when used right and regularly. We all know that to maintain a following, you must post frequently with engaging photos and conversation starters. As I said before, if I didn't have a publishing tool, I probably wouldn't post.

I tested multiple free platforms. They were clunky, complicated, and honestly, a complete waste of time. When I finally broke down and purchased Publer, I was shocked at its easy use. It was relatively low cost for the incredible time savings it offered. Needless to say, this is another service that has saved a lot of time. It isn't something I would invest in until you have a steady flow of funding, but once you get going, it is well worth it.

No matter what form of communication you use, social media, text messages, or email, you must remember how short people's attention spans are and how lazy their eyes are. Your writing must have plenty of white space and use bold text to provide emphasis. Include plenty of breaks in the text, and include graphics to assist in taking it to the next level.

Using graphics to draw attention to key points can distinguish between someone blowing past your comments or stopping just long enough to pique their interest. Thankfully, with the vast array of tech available today, it is easy to do this for free or very cheaply.

I use Canva because the templates and sharing capabilities make it incredibly easy. They offer a free version with loads of options and minimal functional limitations. The paid version of Canva allows you to add team members to share the responsibilities.

You are one person, and you can't do it all. Creating a team on Canva where you all can work and share information and ideas, along with your brand colors and styles, is BRILLIANT. There have even been times when we work on designs together from across the state in real time!

I feel silly grazing over some of those things. It might be common knowledge for many people, especially the younger crowd. However, these are the things that I had to learn on the fly. I spent a lot of time figuring out how to do such basic things and why they are essential, time I could have spent on actual activism or with my family. I hope you find that this has provided you with a place to start and makes your journey easier.

I will continue to offer crash courses for those who want to learn more about writing style, graphic design, and more. I have included all the links and resources on my website wtajourney.com/rnbook, where you can access them easily. Use what benefits you and leave the rest.

I have included referral links for the different services I have discussed. I genuinely use these platforms for my organization and have found success. I will not promote something that I don't use and LOVE.

If you decide to go with any of these vendors, I would appreciate it if you use my referral links. It is one way you can help feed my mission to resuscitate nursing and continue to add helpful resources for you as you heal our profession. If you don't want to use them, that's ok too.

I believe in process improvement and constantly questioning the status quo. So, if you find helpful alternatives, please feel free to reach out and let me know. Technology and services change so fast that it would be impossible to keep up on my own.

With all that being said, infrastructure isn't glamorous, but it's what separates movements that fizzle from the ones that make history. The tools and tactics you build now will either buy back your time or bleed it dry later. Don't wait until things get chaotic to set up your systems.

Do it now, while you're still building. Because once the pressure hits, your structure is what will carry the weight. And if you've done it right, it won't just carry you, it will multiply you.

I wish you the best in building your foundation and the impending success of resuscitating nursing.

10
You Were Built For This

"Rather, ten times, die in the surf,
heralding the way to a new world,
than stand idly on the shore."
– Florence Nightingale

Let's get real for a moment.

If you've made it this far in the book, reading about political fights, strategic mobilization, organizational structure, and public confrontation, you ARE ready to fight... However, you might also feel a pit in your stomach.

It could be fear.
It could be relief.
It could be a sense of overwhelm.
Maybe a touch of exhilaration and adrenaline?

If you are like me, it could all of that plus a voice in the back of your mind whispering,

"What if I screw this up?
What if I am not good enough?
What if I lose my job?
What if I can't handle the pressure?"

Every single leader who has stepped into this kind of fight has felt the sting of that same voice. I have heard it more times than I can count.

These feelings are not a sign that you are unqualified. They are a sign that you understand precisely how big the fight is and how high the stakes are.

It is confirmation that you are standing on the edge of greatness.

You are about to resuscitate nursing.

I would be worried if you didn't feel a little trepidation. You should feel the weight of this because it is monumental.

That twinge means you're the kind of leader who won't take this responsibility lightly.
You will act with integrity.
You stand in morality.
You force ethical behavior.

But here's the truth that fear, self-doubt, and anxiety want to hide from you:

You were built for this.

You are a nurse. When lives are literally seconds away from ending, you perform miracles. Sure, you went to nursing school, but that didn't prepare you for everything, did it? You bear the weight of critical decisions while exhausted, under-resourced, and often unappreciated. You navigate human complexity, grief, and suffering every single shift. It wasn't just your schooling that got you where you are today. You have the grit, the heart, and the moral backbone this profession requires.

Now, you're being asked to bring those same skills to the larger arena, where the health of your profession and your patients are at stake.

Did you let fear stop your first IV?
Your first solo assignment?

What about the first time you ran a code?
No, you didn't.

By reading this book, you have already gotten a load of training. Now it is time for one more integral piece, understanding how to protect yourself while you fight. This has been sprinkled throughout the book, so we will wrap up a few key pieces in the next section.

Remember: Nurses don't let fear freeze them out. Nurses take the next step in spite of the odds.

You were built to resuscitate nursing!

Protect Yourself While Leading the Fight

Legal Tips for Leaders

I need to start with the obligatory disclaimer. **This is not legal advice.** I am not an attorney. I highly encourage you to follow up with a qualified attorney.

Think of this more as the warning light on the IV pump, like the one that flashes yellow or orange before it decides there is an occlusion.

Get informed, get counsel, and stay protected. Here are four areas I want to touch on: knowing your rights, whistleblower protections, defamation, and employment boundaries.

Know Your Rights

We live in America and have the First Amendment right to freedom of speech. You have the right to speak out about matters of public concern, especially regarding patient safety, working conditions, and healthcare policy. That does not mean there won't be any consequences. The First Amendment means they can't stop you, but it doesn't mean they can't fire you.

As we discussed in Chapter Eight, you have some protection under the National Labor Relations Act to conduct **"concerted activity"**. That simply means two or more staff members discussing conditions and the need for corrective action.

As with most things in life, these rules are not all-encompassing. Taking these actions **off the clock** can provide more protection and keep you from facing disciplinary actions. If you are speaking publicly, it is advisable to make a disclaimer similar to:

"These thoughts are my own and do not reflect those of my employer or other affiliations."

This is not a "get out of jail free card," but it may help prevent legal action. Make sure you discuss the specifics with your attorney. The same goes for whistleblower protection. Some people think they protect everyone who does the right thing. That is not the case.

Whistleblower Protections

They Vary By State. Know Yours!

If you think you will automatically be protected for speaking out as a whistleblower, you better think again.

While there are limited federal whistleblower protections, each state has its own laws, which vary considerably. I know the word "whistleblower" has become trendy, and I don't want that to become your downfall.

Just because you saw a nurse on TikTok claiming to be a whistleblower doesn't mean she received any protection. I have known several over the years, many of whom lost their jobs and more.

Not all employees are protected in every state. For example, in some states, like where I live in Indiana, you don't have protection unless you use federal protections or are a public (government) employee.

State law will dictate:

- **Who is protected**
- **Where issues must be reported**
- **What kinds of reports will be accepted**
- **Whether you will receive any protection from retaliation**

Shockingly, in some states, reports of unsafe staffing and ethical concerns may not be protected unless they concern a specific law, regulation, or an obvious patient risk.

Understanding your state's laws and keeping impeccable documentation of the issues will be your safeguard. **Consulting with an attorney before going public is the best course of action.**

It doesn't end there, though. You can still use the tactics in this book to rally staff, patients, and others to force change, even without official whistleblower protections. The benefit may be that you aren't gagged by court order until the courts can settle things.

Understand Defamation, Slander, and Retaliation

First of all, **keep the receipts**, not only for what the politicians say, but *for the things you say.*

If you are speaking at an event, ensure you can provide sources of information. Be sure that what you are saying is not a matter of opinion or speculation, but of fact.

If you are asked a question and you are unsure of the answer, **don't guess. Don't speculate. Don't wing it.** If you do, these moments will come back to haunt you.

Bottom line: *If you can't prove it, don't say it.*

This will help protect you from "accidental" defamation. If it feels like gossip, don't do it. If you wonder if you should say it, don't. Stay sharp and on point with facts.

Even if you do everything right, you may still face retaliation via demotion, disciplinary actions, or even harassment.

If you start to feel like things are off:
Document. Document. Document.

You will act like the scribe in a code: Names, times, descriptions, everyone in the room, the whole shebang! This documentation can be a life raft when things get rough.

You may also want to consult with your attorney to find out if your state is a **single-party state**. Being a single-party state means that you can record audio as long as one person on the recording (you) knows it is being recorded.

That would mean it could be admissible in court as long as you knew you were recording. **Also, check your employer's policies.** Some employers prohibit recordings even if your state law allows them. Violating those policies can still get you fired, even if it wouldn't get you sued. Follow up with your attorney to determine where the lines are and the risks and benefits associated with each.

If you have made recordings before consulting with an attorney, keep that fact to yourself until you can speak with one specializing in employment or whistleblower cases. Ensure recordings are secured to prevent accidental release. Even if you don't release them, you could still face repercussions.

If you cannot record, things can quickly become a game of he said, she said. Such claims don't hold up well in court.

What I have been encouraged to do is to follow conversations, meetings, and other exchanges via email:

"Hi Susie,

I wanted to follow up after our meeting (date) to ensure I understood everything correctly. (Insert narrative.)

Please reply clarifying if needed or confirming that we have the same understanding."

An email like this can help you document what was said and outline the next steps to proceed. Simply sending and receiving emails is not enough. You must secure the documentation. Ensure you print them and/or send copies to your personal account.

I always save them in one folder, the "Red Rover Folder", because as soon as you receive communication or complete documentation, *Red Rover, Red Rover, send it right over.* This way, you have **chronological documentation.**

Know Your Employment Boundaries

That brings us to the final aspect, knowing your employment boundaries.

We've already touched on much of this, but it is worth reviewing.

First, don't use company equipment, technology, or products when resuscitating nursing.

That means no email, no computers, and no phones. No printers, no paper, no supplies. Keep it separate. Do not give your employer any reason to fire you.

That makes this next one obvious: **don't use company time to work on advocacy.**

If you are on the clock, that is their time. If you are paid for breaks, I would be leery of using them.

If your lunch is unpaid, that is YOUR time. But if your 15-minute breaks are paid… PAUSE. I would be very cautious.

Think about it. You would have no way to prove you were on your unpaid 15-minute break while sitting at the nurse's desk searching for "political activism" or other keywords they could use against you. Be smart about how, when, and where you work.

Bottom line:
You are about to enter a fight where your adversaries will look for any angle to discredit or silence you.

Remember, this is not legal advice. Think of this as that yellow light on the IV pump letting you know what traps lie in wait.

Consult with an attorney, so you don't need one, kinda like pulling the death packet, so if the terminal patient passes away at the end of your shift, everything is ready. A little bit of prep is totally worth it.

Besides, when done right, **resuscitating nursing is worth the work!**

Where to Go from Here: Practical Next Steps

Now that you have the foundational education, here is where I would suggest you begin:

If you purchased the workbook along with this book, you may have already started and been working through the steps one by one as we went along. If so, you are already ahead of the class. Keep it up!

If not, that is ok. Either go purchase one on Amazon or download the resources now.

You can find them on wtajourney.com/rnbook and put what you have learned to good use by getting to work.

Pick a battle. Start small if you must, but start. Choose an issue you can win or an area where you can build momentum and dive in.

Gather your receipts. Begin documenting, even if you're not ready to act yet. You will need them.

Find a mentor. Someone outside your immediate fight who can help you see clearly when things get tough.

Build your army. Start with a simple petition, an email list, or even a text group. You need people. No movement wins alone.

Protect your list. Keep your contacts secure. Never hand them over.

Educate yourself on your state's laws. As we covered in the Legal Tips, knowledge is a form of protection.

Begin building a small team. Even one or two committed allies will change what you can accomplish.

Stay rooted in your mission. Scope creep will be your enemy, pulling you in too many directions. Stay focused.

And most of all: Begin.

Despite years in activism, there are times when I still feel like I am simply taking the next right step. Advocacy is tough, and you won't always have the answers.

The best leaders are forged in action, not in waiting.

Building Forward: Movement and Legacy

This moment right here. This is a pivotal point.

It feels a little like standing at the edge of the ocean. You're watching the waves come in, some small and lapping gently at your feet, inviting you to step in. The moment you do, you feel the strength of the water beneath the surface, the way it pulls the sand out from under your feet and draws you further in.

That's where you are now.

You're feeling the pull. You've read the lessons, sharpened your skills, and learned how to protect yourself. You're standing on the edge of something much larger than yourself, and that next step can feel both thrilling and intimidating.

You may be thinking, *This is a lot. Do I really want to step this far in?*

It's a fair question. The truth is, not everyone will take the next step.

Many people will read this book, nod in agreement, and put it down. They will convince themselves they're too busy, that someone else will take the lead, or that they'll get involved "when the timing is better."

That time never comes… and neither do improvements.

But you are not "everyone."

You've come this far because you know in your gut that the time will never be perfect. The system is broken now. Nurses are burning out now. Patients are suffering now. And no one in leadership has any intention of fixing it.

Don't be fooled, here's the real beauty of this moment:

We are the ones who have the power to turn it all around.

We are the ones who will breathe life back into our profession.

We are the ones who will build a legacy that the "Lady with the Lamp" would be proud of.

Florence Nightingale once said, *"Rather, ten times, die in the surf, heralding the way to a new world, than stand idly on the shore."*

That is the mindset we must carry forward.

No excuses. No waiting. No, leaving it to someone else.

The longer we wait, the more work there will be to do. We can't afford to put this off any longer.

You must decide, will you wait for permission? Will you wait for perfection?

Florence Nightingale didn't. Why should you?

You don't need every answer. You need to start. If you don't, your legacy will never have a chance to form.

The work of advocacy is not glamorous. It is often exhausting. It will test your patience, your resilience, and sometimes your relationships. But it will also sharpen you. It will connect you with others willing to carry the lamp.

And when you get discouraged, and you will, remember this:

You are on a journey unlike any you could imagine. A journey that will lead to meaningful change and into a metaphorical lamp that other nurses can use to light their way.

This is legacy work.

Every nurse who stands up today changes what is possible for the next generation of nurses. Every win you achieve, every conversation you change, every piece of truth you bring into the light matters, not just for today's patients, but for the patients and nurses who will come after us.

Legacy is the real reward. Not a headline. Not a handshake from a politician.

Your legacy is a healthcare system that is once again worthy of the trust patients place in it, because nurses refused to let it wither away.

And that is why you must be relentless. Because they will count on your exhaustion, they will take advantage of you. They will count on your division. They will hope you will burn out and go away.

Do not give them that satisfaction.

Pace yourself. Surround yourself with others who carry the same light. Use the tools in this book to build a movement that can withstand storms and outlive any single leader.

Resuscitating nursing will not be easy, but it is necessary. And there is no one better equipped than you.

Call to Action

If you plan on or even think you might be in this fight to resuscitate nursing for more than a year or two, I encourage you to start fundraising.

I can't help but laugh at that statement, "be in this fight for more than a year or two."

When I started activism, I thought I could whip my issue into shape in five years and then move on to healthcare reform.

My initial issue is not "whipped into shape." I will be fighting in that arena for years to come. However, it just dawned on me that my aspiration of taking on healthcare reform has come to fruition. It has not come to be through my own activism, but by sharing this knowledge with you.

God willing, this will leave a far greater impact than my individual activism.

Here is what I want you to remember as you close this book:

Every action you take from now on will either breathe life back into a profession gasping under the weight of broken systems or add to the crushing weight of bureaucracy.

You were **not** called to be passive in the face of injustice.

You were **not** called to watch nursing fade away while politicians and corporate interests profit.

You were **not** called to bear witness to preventable harm without taking action.

You were built for this.

You have walked into more codes, faced more impossible moments, and carried more moral weight than most people ever will.

Do not underestimate what you have been prepared to do.

Nurses are the moral center of healthcare.
Without us, the system collapses.
Without our voices, patients suffer in silence.
Without our leadership, bad actors win.

Do not wait for tomorrow.

Grab your workbook. (See details on page 202.)

Use the tools.

Lay down your foundation. Build your army. Pick your battles. Grow your team. Mobilize them.

Start NOW.

The work will be long. The wins will sometimes be slow.

But this is legacy work. We are creating something that Florence Nightingale would be proud of.

Much like her work, what we do now will change care for generations of nurses who will follow us and the innumerable patients they will serve.

Stand tall.

Carry your lamp high to spread and share the light.

Resuscitate nursing.

Appendix: Referenced Materials

This list includes materials and sources referenced throughout the book. It is intended to provide context, support further research, and promote continued learning.

- Get all the resources in this book: wtajourney.com/rnbook
- Learn more about moral injury: wajourney.com/mip
- Find your nurse practice act: www.ncsbn.org/npa
- *Confrontational Politics* by HL Richardson, (1993).
- 2025 ANA Code of Ethics for Nurses: American Nurses Association. (2025). *Code of Ethics for Nurses* [ebook edition]. Nursesbooks. ISBN 9781963052244 https://codeofethics.ana.org/provisions
- The Joint Commission: https://www.jointcommission.org/
- Internal Revenue Service: https://www.irs.gov/charities-non-profits
- National Labor Relations Board: https://www.nlrb.gov/

Affiliate links

If you choose to use one of the vendors I have discussed, please use my referral links. *If you purchase through these links, I may earn a commission at no additional cost to you.* Most give some sort of incentive to you, too!

- Texting - Project Broadcast: http://www.projectbroadcast.com/?afmc=35s (Rotating referral bonuses. May include free credits)
- Donation Platforms - Donorbox: https://donorbox.org/orgs/new?grsf=8wtheu (Use this link and get a $50 gift card after raising $100)

- Social Media Schedulers:
  Publer: https://publer.com/wtajourney
  (Save %5 by using this link)

Resuscitating Nursing Workbook & Field Manual

Available on Amazon.

This *Workbook & Field Manual* is your hands-on guide to turning insight into impact.

This isn't just a collection of reflection questions.

It's a strategic tool built for nurses who are ready to lead the charge at the bedside, in boardrooms, and beyond.

Inside you'll find:

- Step-by-step worksheets to identify, triage, and target the most urgent problems in your facility or community.
- Proven frameworks to build a team, craft messaging, and sustain pressure for success.
- Mobilization planning tools—petitions, campaign scripts, diamond formation tactics, and more.
- Tactical pages for documenting political commitments, tracking infrastructure, and choosing the right legal structure for your advocacy.
- Prompts designed to challenge your mindset, clarify your "why," and prepare you for real-world resistance.

Whether you're just starting out or already have an army, this workbook transforms the big ideas in *Resuscitating Nursing* into actionable steps.

We are Resuscitating Nursing.

About the Author

Ashley Grogg, MSN-RN, BC-FMP, is a nurse, educator, and reformer with a fierce devotion to integrity in healthcare. Born and raised on a family farm in rural Indiana, Ashley learned early that hard work, faith, and personal responsibility weren't just values, they were a lifestyle. After watching her own family navigate severe health crises with vastly different outcomes, she made a vow: every patient would be treated like family.

Ashley spent over a decade in acute care and the insurance industry, excelling in patient education and outcome improvement. As medicine shifted toward protocols and profit margins, she grew heartbroken, witnessing how profits exceeded patient well-being and safety. In 2018, she walked away from traditional healthcare and founded *Wellness Through Awareness*, a private consulting practice that empowers individuals to reclaim their health through informed decision-making, education, and personalized support.

Today, Ashley is a bold advocate for transparency, patient rights, and ethical reform. Her work in grassroots policy reflects a deep belief that everyday citizens, especially nurses, are the key to transforming broken systems. She speaks with the clarity of a clinician and the courage of one unbound from earthly fears.

Ashley lives in Indiana with her husband, Charles, and their four daughters, whom they homeschool with the same conviction she brings to every part of her life: that faith, truth, liberty, and compassion will always matter.

Resuscitating Nursing is her charge to the brave, those willing to reject complacency, lead with conviction, and breathe life back into the heart of nursing.

www.ingramcontent.com/pod-product-compliance
Lightning Source LLC
LaVergne TN
LVHW050816061126
851857LV00012B/828

Resuscitating Nursing